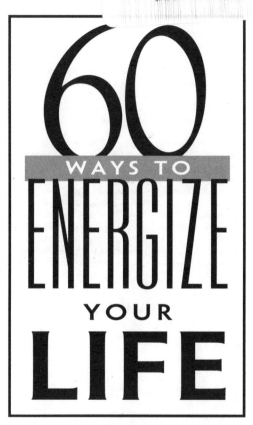

# 60
## WAYS TO
# ENERGIZE
## YOUR
# LIFE

Compiled by
**Jan W. Kuzma, Kay Kuzma, and DeWitt S. Williams**

REVIEW AND HERALD® PUBLISHING ASSOCIATION
HAGERSTOWN, MD 21740

Scripture quotations marked NASB are from the *New American Standard
Bible*, © The Lockman Foundation 1960, 1962, 1963, 1968, 1971, 1972,
1973, 1975, 1977.

Texts credited to NEB are from *The New English Bible*. © The Delegates of
the Oxford University Press and the Syndics of the Cambridge University
Press 1961, 1970. Reprinted by permission.

Texts credited to NIV are from the *Holy Bible, New International Version*.
Copyright © 1973, 1978, 1984, International Bible Society. Used by permission of Zondervan Bible Publishers.

Texts credited to NKJV are from The New King James Version. Copyright
© 1979, 1980, 1982, Thomas Nelson, Inc., Publishers.

Texts credited to REB are from *The Revised English Bible*. Copyright © Oxford
University Press and Cambridge University Press, 1989. Reprinted by permission.

Bible texts credited to RSV are from the Revised Standard Version of the Bible,
copyright © 1946, 1952, 1971, by the Division of Christian Education of the
National Council of the Churches of Christ in the U.S.A. Used by permission.

Verses marked TLB are taken from *The Living Bible*, copyright © 1971
Tyndale House Publishers, Wheaton, Ill. Used by permission.

This book was
Edited by Gerald Wheeler and Richard W. Coffen
Copyedited by Jocelyn Fay and James Cavil
Cover design by GenesisDesign/Bryan Gray
Typeset: 10.5/12 Goudy

PRINTED IN U.S.A.

05 04          7 6 5

**R&H Cataloging Service**
60 ways to energize your life. Compiled by
    Jan W. Kuzma, Kay Kuzma, and DeWitt S. Williams.

    1. Health.   I. Kuzma, Jan W., comp.   II. Kuzma, Kay, comp.
III. Williams, DeWitt S., comp.

                         613
ISBN 0-8280-1411-6

# CONTENTS

# The Miracle Bean

*Every good endowment and every perfect gift is from above, coming down from the Father of lights with whom there is no variation or shadow due to change. James 1:17, RSV.*

Webster defines a miracle as "an extraordinary event manifesting divine intervention in human affairs." Usually we think of miracles as events that are beyond our limited human understanding of the natural world. They inspire awe and bring us to our knees in the humbling presence of God's power and mercy, such as during a spontaneous healing of a life-threatening disease.

But most of us recognize that even some easily explained, everyday occurrences so reflect God's goodness and magnificence that they contain a touch of the miraculous. No matter that science explains their occurrence. They still take our breath away and fill us with awe just the same, whether it be the cry of a newborn baby or a perfect rainbow.

But some miracles seem to escape our notice because we don't look hard enough or we forget that God's gifts to us are not always earth-shattering.

Nutritionists who study plant-based diets have found such a "miracle." Soybeans are rich in the highest quality protein. Inexpensive and easy to grow, they produce 20 times more protein an acre than an acre devoted to raising beef. So versatile is the soybean that in one form or another it appears in nearly every kind of dish imaginable. Packaged in this little bean is a host of natural substances that have impressive health protective effects, earning soy the nickname "miracle bean." Scientists have found in soybeans substances called isoflavones, which appear in no other commonly consumed food. Isoflavones have been linked to a reduced risk for cancer, heart disease, and osteoporosis.

A miracle? Webster might not agree that soybeans meet the strictest definition of that word. But God's people know that the true miracle is His never-ending desire to bless us with gifts for our welfare and happiness. Each of these gifts is a miraculous sign of His great love for us. They come in big and small packages, and often escape our notice. But our lives are enriched when we recognize and are grateful for each gift—whether it be healing, a baby, a rainbow, or a little brown bean.

MARK AND VIRGINIA MESSINA

*Lord, teach me to see the many gifts with which You bless my life, and to be always thankful for all the good things You provide.*

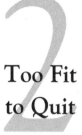

# Too Fit
# to Quit

*Let the morning bring me word of your unfailing love, for I have put my trust in you. Show me the way I should go, for to you I lift up my soul. Ps. 143:8, NIV.*

There's no great accomplishment just in living many years," said an active 91-year-old. "Nursing homes are filled with medicated survivors—as if that has to be the fate of those who reach old age. But to live to those ages and still be independent, physically active, and mentally alert, that is an accomplishment."

And that's exactly what Charlotte Hamlin has been doing as she sets walking and cycling records across the country. "The closer we live by the laws of nature," she says, "the better we will feel and the longer we will live." And what are the laws of nature? According to Charlotte, the secret's in the acronym FRESH START: Fresh air, Rest, Exercise, Sunshine, Happiness, Simple diet, The use of water, Abstemiousness, Restoration, and Trust in divine power.

Charlotte, nearing her eightieth birthday, cycles

from 50 to 80 miles a day and has proved to millions that we can stay productive and healthy at any age. From 1973 until she retired in 1986 she organized and directed a summer health-screening program, and founded the three C's, a risk evaluation program that tested for potential risk for coronaries, cancer, and CVA (stroke).

In 1986 Charlotte retired as assistant professor of nursing at Andrews University and established Fresh Start, a health-conditioning live-in program. When she was 68 she and her son, Gene, formed a non-profit organization, Global Trek International.

The same year she walked and cycled from coast to coast, leaving southern California in March 1987 and arriving 67 days later at Charleston, South Carolina. She made a 32-day trek across Europe that fall. The following year her 9,000 miles of pedaling took her through portions of Israel, Pakistan, India, Thailand, China, Japan, Guam, and Hawaii, and she finished at her birthplace in Canada on her seventieth birthday.

An article about Charlotte carried the title "Too Fit to Quit." Not a bad slogan as she pedals around the world, reminding us that God has a work for us to do, regardless of our age.

JAN W. AND KAY KUZMA

*What could you be doing to help you earn the slogan "Too Fit to Quit"?*

# Cure Worry With a Song

*Therefore I tell you, do not worry about your life, what you will eat; or about your body, what you will wear. Life is more than food, and the body more than clothes. Luke 12:22, 23, NIV.*

J. C. Penney, the genius behind one of the world's largest chains of department stores, had built his business to a multimillion-dollar level when he lost $40 million in the crash of 1929. Three years later, when he was 56 years of age, he had to sell out to satisfy his creditors, leaving him virtually broke. He worried so much that he couldn't sleep. The stress from his chronic fatigue depressed his immune system, and he suffered a relapse of the chicken pox virus that had been dormant in his nerves since he had had the rash as a child. The recurrence of this virus, called shingles, causes severe pain. He was hospitalized at the Battle Creek Sanitarium and given sedatives, but he still tossed and turned all night. Broken physically and mentally, he was overwhelmed with a fear of death and wrote farewell letters to his wife and son, since he didn't expect to live until morning.

Then he awoke to the staff singing in the hospital chapel, "Be not dismayed whate'er betide, God will take care of you . . ." Following the music to its source, he slipped into a back row. Mr. Penney said something happened at that moment that he couldn't explain. "I felt as if I had been instantly lifted out of the darkness of a dungeon into warm, brilliant sunlight. I felt the power of God as I had never felt it before. I realized that I alone was responsible for all my troubles. I knew that God with His love was there to help me. From that day to this, my life has been free from worry. I am 71 years old, and the most dramatic and glorious minutes of my life were those I spent in that chapel that morning."

As a result of the renewing of J. C. Penney's mind through the power of a song, he went on to rebuild his financial empire to well over the billion-dollar mark and celebrated with his family and friends his ninety-fifth birthday.

JAN W. AND KAY KUZMA

*When you're tempted to worry, what song could you think of or sing to relieve the stress?*

# God's Gift
# of Time

*Remember the Sabbath day by keeping it holy. Six days you shall labor and do all your work, but the seventh day is a Sabbath to the Lord your God. Ex. 20:8-10, NIV.*

I n our high-tech, stress-filled, busy world of work we need a weekly, 24 hours of downtime. We need to rest from the overstimulation of our body's adrenal system, the root of many modern stress problems. That's why God gave us the Sabbath. "The Sabbath was made for man, not man for the Sabbath" (Mark 2:27, NIV). People were to work for six days and rest for one—a rhythm that history has shown to fit human life.

People have tried other rhythms. For instance, in 1793 the French adopted a calendar of 12 months of 30 days each. Workers stayed on the job for nine days and rested on the tenth. Soon, though, they discontinued that calendar as unworkable because workers didn't want to work nine days before getting a day of rest.

During World War II the United States and Great Britain speeded up the production of war materials.

Many factories went to 74-hour workweeks. Before long they realized that their employees were averaging only 66 hours of actual work. These same factory workers complained about feeling irritable. Morale dropped. Accidents increased. Spoilage soared.

Factory owners soon decreased the workweek. In the United States some factories added more workers and others introduced three eight-hour shifts instead of increasing the hours of the single shift. What were the results? They had higher production, fewer spoiled items, lower rates of absenteeism, and better morale.

In Great Britain when they reduced the number of working hours to 48 a week (eight-hour days, six days a week), production went up. The British then went so far as to declare a mandatory rest of one day each week and gave their workers two weeks of annual vacation.

The idea of resting one full day out of every seven is as old as the beginning of the human race. It was God's gift to the human race to preserve life and health. Isn't it about time we enjoyed God's gift of time?

JAN W. KUZMA AND CECIL MURPHY

*How can you reap the health benefits from the Sabbath day as God intended?*

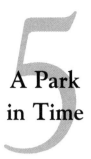

# A Park
# in Time

*He [Jesus] went to Nazareth, where he had been brought up, and on the Sabbath day he went into the synagogue, as was his custom. And he stood up to read. . . . "He has sent me to proclaim freedom for the prisoners and recovery of sight for the blind, to release the oppressed." Luke 4:16-18, NIV.*

**A** *park is a refuge in space.* My friends who live in Manhattan tell me how precious Central Park is to them. They live and work surrounded by towering buildings and pavement. The pace of city life is frantic, unrelenting. But when they step into Central Park, everything changes. Trees offer shade. They find grass for spreading a blanket and sharing a picnic. My friends say that while in the park they feel a thousand miles away from the pressure, the stress, the frantic pace.

*The Sabbath is a refuge in time.* For 24 hours every week God invites us to put aside the struggle to earn a living, to get A's in school, to keep an immaculate house. During those 24 hours He invites us to act out the rest we have in Jesus. The Sabbath is the gospel in dramatic form. For a whole day we rest in the accomplishments of our Saviour. We shut out all the demands and expectations of the world and luxuriate in the promises of God.

Notice how Jesus kept the Sabbath (Luke 4). During a Sabbath worship service Jesus quoted from Isaiah 61, a passage that predicts the coming of the Messiah in the language of the Jubilee, the time when Israelites should release captives and set free the oppressed (Lev. 25:10, 40, 54).

Luke then follows with two healing episodes. Both of them occurred on Sabbath. The first one happened in Capernaum during a Sabbath service at which Jesus healed a possessed man, freeing him from spiritual slavery to a demon (Luke 4:33-37). The second occurred later the same day in the home of Peter, where Jesus and the disciples had gone to eat after church. There Jesus healed Peter's mother-in-law's high fever (verses 38, 39).

Notice the way Luke tells these stories. First Jesus announces His mission as Messiah by quoting Isaiah about freeing the oppressed. Next He brings spiritual healing to a man possessed by a demon. Then He gives physical healing to a woman suffering from a fever. I think Jesus was telling us something about the meaning of the Sabbath, don't you?

LONNIE MELASHENKO

*Why do you spend all your time among towering problems and dead-end pavement, when God has provided a weekly park in time for you to enjoy? Why not follow the custom of Jesus?*

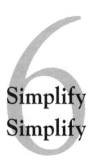

# Simplify
## Simplify

*Whosoever believeth in him should not perish, but have everlasting life. John 3:16.*

**S**everal years ago I joined a group on a 10-day backpacking trip across the Sierra Nevada range. Everything we needed—food, clothes, cooking equipment, tent—had to fit in our backpack. Since the recommended load for a backpack is one third your body weight, I needed to keep mine below 60 pounds.

I had been on several weekend hikes before, but packing for 10 days is a far cry from packing for two days. I had to keep reminding myself to simplify. No fancy meals—only freeze-dried entrées that mix with boiled water. Not two coats to change into—just one. Not three pairs of pants—just the one pair to wear. Not six sets of underwear—just two. No extra shoes or towels. No books for evening reading. Every item had to pass the test: "Do I *really* need this item?" A friend of mine even cut off the handle of his toothbrush to eliminate excess weight. What a difference it all made while hiking on the trail. Every pound we left behind was a blessed relief those 10 days.

At times in my life I thought salvation was too complicated—at least the way some make it appear. It seemed as if reaching heaven depended on what I ate, how I dressed, where I went, how I interpreted Bible prophecy, how I chose to worship, and on and on. The simple formula of John 3:16 had become a 100-pound backpack.

But Jesus set the record straight. In a stern rebuke, He declared: "Woe to you, teachers of the law and Pharisees, you hypocrites! You shut the kingdom of heaven in men's faces. You yourselves do not enter, nor will you let those enter who are trying to" (Matt. 23:13, 14, NIV).

Simplify! Simplify! Salvation is not so complicated. The prophet Micah reduced it to three simple elements: "To do justly, to love mercy, and to walk humbly with your God" (Micah 6:8, NKJV). Ah! Now that's a load off my shoulders.

LARRY RICHARDSON

*How could you simplify your life so the load you are carrying doesn't weigh you down?*

# Grief: An Experience in Learning and Leaning

*Those who know your name will trust in you, for you, Lord, have never forsaken those who seek you. Ps. 9:10, NIV*

**W**hen my father passed away two years ago, I was angry with God. Why did it have to be my father? There were other fathers He could take; why mine? I felt God had deserted me. Who was going to look after me? Who was going to help me provide funding for my school fees? Who was going to stand beside me through my adolescence? Who was going to teach me how to change my car oil? Who would give me away when I got married?

On Father's Day I had no reason to go to the Hallmark store for a card. Neither would I have any reason to go to the men's department store for a gift. Most of all, I missed having my father around and was furious with God. I couldn't face the world alone! Why me? I wondered.

Jesus asked God, when He was nailed to the cross, why God had forsaken Him: "Eli, Eli, lama sabachthani? that is to say, My God, my God, why hast thou forsaken me?" (Matt. 27:46). And I asked the same question.

These past two years have been a learning and leaning experience. Learning that God allows trials and tribulations to attack us so that if we choose to let God help us, we can be stronger. And it's been a leaning experience. In God I have found my solitude, peace, and hope. God has not forsaken me. He has always been my friend and partner.

I began reading the Psalms, because David had many of the same doubts I had. He could tell God exactly how he was feeling, get it out of his system, and turn around and praise God. I've learned that that is the answer to getting rid of the bitterness and finding healing. And the result is an intimacy with God that I never had before.

Currently I am working with hospice patients. I have had the opportunity to share my experiences with my patients and their families. God is using my personal experience to help my faith and be a witness for Him. And I can praise Him for that.

BARBARA CHOO

*Have you been feeling that God has forsaken you? Tell God how you're feeling, read His Word, and experience His healing.*

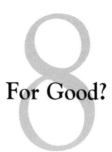

# For Good?

*And we know that all things work together for good to them that love God, to them who are the called according to his purpose.* Rom. 8:28.

**N**one of us ever planned our lives exactly as they are. But real life is never packed in neat boxes with labels to be unloaded at the end of the journey like the contents of a moving van. Our second son, Terry, has a wheelchair, which we call his "purple Porsche," so he can keep up with the rest of us.

Terry has been part of our family for 25 years. Years of love, hope, tears, joys, frustration—as well as lessons in patience and dependence that have slowed us, his family, down.

My morning prayer for "strength just for today" has become so natural, I can't imagine beginning the day any other way. For having a person with a long-term disability in one's family is an everyday challenge, not just once a month or for a weekend. And God's strength has sustained us all, daily, weekly, monthly throughout those 25 years.

The word "good" and "for good" are poles apart.

God's original plan did not include families having sons or daughters with disabilities. Having such a son or daughter is not "good," but personal reactions to circumstances can work "for good" when God's children allow Him to mold us despite less than perfect circumstances. For God waits patiently, His arms outstretched toward His hurting children, desiring to be their comforter, their strength, and their guide.

I can understand my own inability to "work my way to heaven" better as I care for my son, doing for him things he cannot do for himself. It reminds me that I cannot be "good enough" for heaven without my Saviour's sacrifice. This fact has transformed my self-sufficient tendencies into grateful acceptance of Jesus' earthly sacrifice.

I look forward to the time when we move from earth to our heavenly mansion, for Terry will be leaving his purple Porsche, and we will enter heaven with our fellow Christians labeled "perfect in Christ." Together we'll walk the golden streets. Memories of the purple Porsche will fade as we, with all heaven's inhabitants, praise God for Christ's death for us that entitles us to our heavenly home.

CONNIE W. NOWLAN

*What are you looking forward to leaving behind when Jesus comes and labels you "perfect in Christ"?*

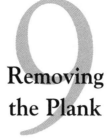

# Removing
the Plank

*Do not judge, or you too will be judged. For in the same way
you judge others, you will be judged. Matt. 7:1, 2, NIV.*

He was just a little guy, barely 6 years old, and
he was afraid. Who wouldn't be with a BB pellet embedded in his eye? Equally fearful were the
young parents, who had rushed him at dusk to our
inner-city emergency department.

As I examined the injured eye, I noted behind
the lower lid an ugly round blot in the delicate mem-
brane, as if someone had poked him with a nail.
Here was the pellet's portal of entry. Somewhere in
the depths lay the errant and malignant sphere of
metal. X-rays could locate it precisely, and perhaps a
skilled eye surgeon would later dissect it out and still
preserve the vision. Maybe.

But first, to complete the examination. As the
mother sat in her corner and sobbed softly and as the
father white-knuckled her hand, I averted the lower
lid. With thumb and finger I sought a better look at
the ugly point of entry. Perhaps I could determine

the direction that the pellet had taken as it bludgeoned its way through the delicate tissue. While comforting my little patient, and holding steady my position, I placed my opposite index finger well below the margin of the lid and squeezed gently. Suddenly, miraculously, the shining metallic orb welled up to the surface, squeezing through the hole and into my eager hand. Placing it on a white square of sterile gauze, I passed it to the happy parents.

BB guns fired indiscriminately at dusk by a careless neighbor boy can be a scourge on defenseless eyes. And removal is rarely so sure or so simple. Yet how easy it is to remove the proverbial mote from a neighbor's eye and fail miserably at finding it in our own! Jesus says, "You hypocrite, first take the plank out of your own eye, and then you will see clearly to remove the speck from your brother's eye" (Matt. 7:5, NIV).

Today let's opt anew for introspection—to see ourselves as others see us, and to refrain from judging others.

RAYMOND O. WEST

*Lord, don't let me be a hypocrite, judging and criticizing others when I have so much in my own life that needs to be cleaned up!*

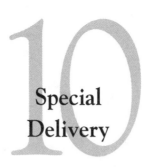

# Special
# Delivery

*In love he predestined us to be adopted as his sons through Jesus Christ, in accordance with his pleasure and will. Eph. 1:4, 5, NIV.*

**D**uring a period of about six years our son begged for a baby sister, even though he knew it would be dangerous for his mother to have any more children. We had mentioned this fact to our cousin, who worked in the labor and delivery unit of a hospital, in case a baby became available for adoption.

Four years passed. We had long forgotten the conversation with the cousin when the phone rang one rainy Sunday afternoon. Our cousin asked if we were still interested in adopting. After we prayed and all agreed, we arranged to meet with the social worker and doctor within the hour.

Within three hours we had decided on a name and were looking at our little pink bundle. Twenty-three hours after the call we had our baby home, while our family and the church family arranged for bottles, blankets, clothing, a car seat, a bassinet, formula, diapers, and even a pediatrician.

Question marks ran through our minds, however: would we love Traci as we did Matthew? Would she respond to us? Would we make it through the adoption process? What if her parents changed their minds? What about Traci's genetic background?

Soon Traci's new daddy knew he couldn't possibly love his little girl more. Her mommy adored her energy and personality, and her brother delighted in holding her and tickling her tummy. Nothing else mattered.

As we've watched Traci respond to our love, we've become more aware of what God has offered us as His adopted children and how deeply hurt He must be when we deny Him.

The God of the universe has said to us: "I will make you my sons and daughters; . . . you shall become members of the royal family and children of the heavenly King" (*Testimonies*, vol. 2, p. 592).

If only we would respond as does little Traci—with utmost love and confidence—and accept the incredible honor of being part of His family. If we choose to be "specially delivered" by Jesus, we can all be adopted heirs of the King, and what heavenly rejoicing that will bring!

ROB, DEBBIE, AND MATTHEW PURVIS

*What does it take to be adopted into God's family? "Come out from among them, and be separate, saith the Lord, and I will receive you, and ye shall be sons and daughters of the Lord Almighty. What a promise!"* (ibid.).

# Being a Trustworthy Envoy

*A wicked messenger falls into trouble, but a trustworthy envoy brings healing. He who ignores discipline comes to poverty and shame, but whoever heeds correction is honored. Prov. 13:17, 18, NIV.*

**B**eing overweight is a major health hazard. You may or may not fall into this category. But all of us have family and friends who do, and their good health is important to us. That's why we must do everything possible to be supportive and encouraging.

Few of us realize that obese people face three times the risk of heart disease, and are four times more likely to have high blood pressure. They also have five times greater risk of developing diabetes, and five times the likelihood of having elevated blood cholesterol.

Furthermore, overweight individuals face six times the chance of developing gallbladder disease, and they will also experience more cancer of the colon, rectum, breast, cervix, uterus, ovaries, and prostate than average-weight people.

But the list of hazards doesn't stop there. Health experts estimate that only 60 percent of obese people reach the age of 60, compared with 90 percent of those who aren't overweight.

A recent survey of Adventists showed that 24 percent considered themselves moderately or considerably overweight. And if you meet one who does, perhaps you can get better acquainted and possibly learn the reason for their condition. Is it their inactive job, their cultural habit of snacking, their lack of moderation, a missing exercise program such as walking, their anxiety or depression that makes them want to eat more than they should? Is it a hereditary problem? Or is it the lack of information and no supportive friends?

Once you get to know them and are a trusted friend, it's easier to provide helpful information or to work together on a weight reduction plan. You must be sympathetic and supportive, not judgmental. The same survey indicates that 76 percent of those overweight are interested in changing their condition, and you may be just the person who will make the critical difference in their lives.

You might not be the good Samaritan who picks up the bloody man on the side of the road, but you can lift up the hope and expectation of someone wanting to get control of their weight problem. Having good support and encouragement is one of the keys for success.

JAN W. KUZMA

*If you fall into the overweight category, seek out supportive friends who can help you keep your commitment to adopt a healthier lifestyle.*

# Time—God's Great Gift

*For in six days the Lord made the heavens and the earth, the sea, and all that is in them, and rested the seventh day. Therefore the Lord blessed the Sabbath day and hallowed it. Ex. 20:11, NKJV.*

**K**nowing that His human children would need time to refresh mind and body after a week of work, at the end of Creation week God prescribed the Sabbath. His prescription still works. Weekly He provides His children time to enjoy His companionship and handiwork.

Our family loves the outdoors, and on Sabbath we take time to bask in God's natural beauty.

Our Sabbath refreshment has included a summer of Sabbath mornings when we watched four baby foxes grow up in the field behind our house. Then one Sabbath afternoon we followed a mother deer and her speckled fawn as they strolled down Lehigh Street, the mother walking protectively between the cars and her baby. Another Sabbath at sunset we watched a beaver eating supper at Rocky Mountain National Park. And one Sabbath a herd of more than 100 elks milled around our jeep, eating and bugling, close enough that we watched without binoculars.

My very favorite Sabbath refreshment took place on the peaceful Moose River in Maine. We took our motored canoe out to a narrow passage and dropped anchor. Sudden movement to our right caught our attention. A family of beavers slid silently into the water and began nibbling twigs and leaves from overhanging branches. A mosquito landed on my nose, and I swatted. A slap of a beaver's tail sent the whole family under-water. We sat motionless, waiting. Then the beavers surfaced and continued with their meal.

Downriver two otters swam toward us, their humped backs rising and falling above the water as they played. As a climax, a deer with a large rack of antlers walked into the water and stood facing us, silhouetted in the sunset colors. Darkness would soon descend, and knowing we had to thread our way through some rocks on the way back to the dock, we reluctantly started the motor. The animals disappeared into the forest. No one can erase from our memories the refreshment that God's gift of time gave us.

And best of all, God's prescription for rest comes every week, not once a year like Christmas. What a wise God!

CONNIE W. NOWLAN

*Take time on the Sabbath to refresh yourself with peaceful scenes of God's creation, and you too will be revitalized.*

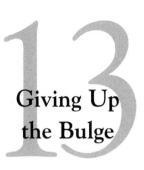

# Giving Up
# the Bulge

*Come to me, all you who are weary and burdened, and I will give you rest. Take my yoke upon you and learn from me, for I am gentle and humble in heart, and you will find rest for your souls. For my yoke is easy and my burden is light. Matt. 11:28-30, NIV.*

**S**ix of us had entered the deep Virginia cave a few hours before on the dangling end of a stout rope. We had ambled, crawled, and crouched our way through tunnels and crawlways from caverns to vast stalactite-strewn rooms. Then we had eaten lunch by the shore of a tiny lake. Yes, it had been a spelunker's day of delights. Somewhere up there on the surface the winter afternoon had waned and it was past time to exit.

Now again, with the aid of our trusty rope, four of our group were already on top. Bob, my stocky spelunker friend, crouched with me on a narrow shelf of solid rock, with 80 feet of dark vertical passageway below and a shaft of wintry light slanting down from above.

Unfortunately, we had a problem—we were stuck just below a narrow confinement. As Bob had clawed his way upward, I had pushed from below.

31

But he was simply too stocky and the defile too narrow. On the way down Bob had been assisted by gravity, but going up, it was like a cork stuck in the neck of a bottle. Several times we had heaved and shoved. Now, breathless and fatigued, we considered our options: a pound of butter for grease? a jackhammer? even a minor earthquake?

In frustration Bob exploded, "You'll just have to leave me here."

With just the breath of a prayer we rallied our strength for a final try. As Bob heaved on the rope, I shoved from below. Nothing! Then, curiously, I noted for the first time a bulge in Bob's back pocket. "Bob," I exulted, "slide back down here and take out your wallet!"

That was it. In our anxiety we'd missed the cause of the jam-up. Bob's wallet had been the plug. With another hefty shove we were soon on top and headed for home.

Concerned over health-related burdens? Why not decide today to give them over to Jesus? Hand Him your anxieties and stress. Trust Him with your empty calories and adipose pounds—and all the rest.

He has promised to make our burdens easy and light.

RAYMOND O. WEST

*What is the bulge in your life that is keeping you from reaching your desired goals? Give it to Jesus and expect a miracle!*

# Sugarcoated Sin

*He [Moses] chose to be mistreated along with the people of God rather than to enjoy the pleasures of sin for a short time. Heb. 11:25, NIV.*

I'll never forget the first time we flew into the poverty-stricken village of Ocoroni, Mexico, to hold a dental clinic. The minute we touched down on that tiny 1,500-foot dirt landing strip more than 100 children ran to the plane, hoping for handouts. When they smiled up at us, my heart sank. Many of them had their front teeth rotted off to the gums because of the habit of sucking on sugarcane.

The children suffered from ignorance and poverty. Sugarcane made them feel good. But they had no one to tell them it was a deceptive pleasure that would end up destroying their teeth, causing them incredible pain and eventual loss.

We could do little with those who flocked to our open shed where we set up our dental clinic but pull teeth. One woman kept trying to move ahead in the line. Through an interpreter we learned that because of the pain she was suffering she had walked 30 miles

(50 kilometers) to get to the clinic, and would have to go back home that day. I pulled 15 of her teeth, each one so rotted down to the gums that I hardly had anything to get a grip on. If only these people had realized the hidden dangers of sugarcane!

Then I thought about the children in my country whose front teeth had begun to rot. Not from sugarcane, but from apple juice, soft drinks, and soda pop given in a bottle from the time they were tiny babies. Some parents didn't know how dangerous it was to allow a child to suck on juice or milk and fall asleep with their teeth literally "sugarcoated." Others, not wanting to put up with a fuss at bedtime if they removed the juice-filled bottle, allowed their innocent children the pleasure that would later result in damaged teeth.

It made me think about how much sin is like sugarcane or the sugar-sweet liquid in a bottle. It tastes good at the time, but without realizing it, we are being destroyed. The pleasures of sin, even for a short time, can have long-lasting and painful consequences.

JERRY MUNCY

*Lord, open my eyes to the hidden dangers of "sugarcoated" sin.*

# Getting Into Biblical Shape

15

*Enoch walked with God; then he was no more, because God took him away. Gen. 5:24, NIV.*

As we look at some of the well-known characters of the Bible, an interesting picture emerges. See Elijah running in front of the horses of Ahab. Imagine David following the sheep mile after mile, and being so physically fit that he could kill a bear with his hands. Picture Abraham trekking about 1,000 miles from Ur of the Chaldees to Canaan on foot. Can you visualize yourself traveling with Jesus as He treads the dusty roads of Palestine? Or follow Paul around on his three missionary journeys?

Do you think you could keep up with any one of these characters if they were to show up today? If not, maybe it's time you got into "biblical shape."

1. *Schedule exercise into your day.* Don't just wait till you "find time" for it. Chances are, you never will.

2. *Exercise frequently*, at least every other day. Daily would be even better.

3. *Enjoy the exercise you choose.* There's no point

35

in trying to improve your body while torturing your mind. Plus, when you exercise with a negative attitude, your body doesn't get as much benefit out of it.

4. *Exercise for at least 30 minutes at a time.*

Exercise can come in many different types, but most people prefer walking. It does wonders for all ages, without the risks involved in more vigorous exercise programs such as jogging or aerobics. Even God walked in the garden of Eden in the cool of the night with Adam and Eve (Gen. 3:8). And Scripture records that centuries later Enoch walked with God.

People who exercise regularly say that it calms their minds and makes them more alert. Perhaps all the walking the Bible greats did was one of the reasons their minds were so perceptive of God's will. They likely spent many hours walking and talking with their Creator. It's a combination that can keep all of us physically as well as spiritually fit. God is eager to bless us, as He did Enoch, Elijah, David, Abraham, Jesus, and Paul, if we will follow their example of maintaining a walking-and-talking-to-Him lifestyle.

NANCY NEWBALL

*What is keeping you from getting out of your chair, stepping out the front door, and walking with the Lord for 30 minutes? God wants you to be physically fit as well as spiritually fit.*

# Breaking an Addictive Habit

*I can do all things through Christ who strengthens me. Phil. 4:13, NKJV.*

**A**gain and again you've tried to quit. You're tired of the guilt that comes from your dependance on food, coffee, sex, pills, cigarettes, alcohol, drugs, or whatever. How can you obtain freedom from your addiction? The following seven steps may be your answer.

**Step 1:** *Exercise.* A brisk walk, a swim, or a bike ride will help by physically removing you from the temptation. Exercise produces endorphins that encourage feelings of optimism and happiness. It gives you energy and relieves the stress that drives you to your habit.

**Step 2:** *Practice positive self-talk.* High self-esteem enables you to see your potential instead of your failures. Remind yourself of your talents and abilities. Stop putting yourself down. When you get up in the morning, look in the mirror and say, "I like myself just the way I am!" (including bulges, hang-ups, and all).

**Step 3:** *Focus on peace of mind.* Turmoil and unrest cause you to revert to your bad habits. A sense of contentment can silence that inner unrest. When you feel upset, read Psalm 23 and focus your thoughts on that green pasture and still water that God has promised you.

**Step 4:** *Accept the fact that you're human and that you may blow it occasionally.* All people have setbacks as they try to break an addictive habit. But feelings of failure lead to guilt and discouragement, which in turn may drive you back to your habit for comfort. It's a vicious cycle, so don't get caught in it. Don't expect yourself to be perfect.

**Step 5:** *Develop an "I can" philosophy.* The ability to break your addictive habit is to a great extent dependent on your attitude. If you truly believe you can do it, you will be more likely to succeed.

**Step 6:** *Develop your power of choice.* Willpower is the best tool to use when trying to break a habitual behavior. It's the ability to say no to something you want and know you shouldn't have.

**Step 7:** *Ask for Jesus' power.* Even though you may have the desire to quit, remember, the power to do so comes from outside yourself. Claim the promise "I can do all things through Christ who strengthens me."

NANCY NEWBALL

*God longs to give you the peace and power you need to change your bad habits. Remember, with God all things are possible.*

# The Breath of Life

*Come near to God and he will come near to you. James 4:8, NIV.*

The day was one of those you dream about. The earth was fresh from the hand of God. "Let us make man in our image" He said (Gen. 1:26, NIV). Bending over, He carefully formed the first human being from the dust of the ground. He lay there. Fragile. Made of dust. There was no movement or life.

God bent again. And He breathed into that dusty form. Air flowed into the being's nose and down into his lungs. It brought life. What joy God must have felt as He witnessed that first breath of His new creature.

Air is the breath of life. We are fully dependent upon it to give us oxygen to operate the powerhouses in our cells. These powerhouses, called mitochondria, are the backbone of every activity carried on in our bodies. They use the oxygen to burn the food that fuels our cells.

There's also an air supply that provides power to

our Christian experience. The power comes from air that's unpolluted by any smog. Martin Luther called this air the "breath of the soul," for just as surely as our physical bodies need air to survive, so our spiritual selves need the power of this air supply to continue to grow. The air that provides such a heavenly atmosphere is prayer.

"*Prayer* is the opening of the heart to God as to a friend. Not that it is necessary in order to make known to God what we are, but in order to enable us to receive Him. Prayer does not bring God down to us, but brings us up to Him" (*Steps to Christ*, p. 93).

God longs to be your friend. He wants you to talk with Him the same way you'd converse with your best friend. The only way you can do that is through prayer. Share your thoughts, your problems, your joys and successes. He listens. The Bible suggests that we should "pray without ceasing" (1 Thess. 5:17). That means becoming so comfortable with the fact that God is our friend that we have a continual open communication with Him. That's when prayer becomes as natural as breathing!

NAD CHURCH MINISTRIES

*Are you looking for a life full of vitality, happiness, and joy? Are you needing a breath of fresh air? Prayer is the air your soul needs to breathe.*

# 18

# The Environment
# and Health

*The nations were angry; and your wrath has come. The time has come . . . for destroying those who destroy the earth. Rev. 11:18, NIV.*

Consider these facts:

• In 1960 the average U.S. citizen produced three pounds of trash per day; today five pounds per person per day go into the trash.

• Ten thousand people die each year from pesticide poisoning, and another 40,000 fall ill. The rapidly increasing use of such chemicals throughout the world threatens water quality and poses risks of increased cancer and birth defects.

• Each year human beings clear an area of tropical forest the size of Scotland; the soil then erodes, the climate begins changing, and the forest's replenishing resources have vanished.

• Scientists estimate that as many as one million species of plant and animal life will have become extinct from the human destruction of forests and ecosystems by the end of the twentieth century.

The beginning of Hosea 4 describes the Lord's

"controversy with the inhabitants of the land" (verse 1). He says that they lack kindness and faithfulness, replacing it with lying, stealing, cheating, adultery, and murder. And what is the result? "The land mourns, and all who live in it waste away" (verse 3, NIV) and the beasts, birds, and even fish disappear.

The Bible clearly laments the deterioration of the environment. When you contrast it with the wondrous pictures of creation's intended harmony and wholeness given in Scripture, you realize that environmental ruin is an offense against God.

At Creation God gave humanity "dominion" over all the earth (Gen. 1:26-28). However, the biblical term *dominion* does not mean arrogant domination. The biblical concept of dominion is connected to two other key ideas—covenant and stewardship. The Bible expresses not only God's covenant with humanity, but also His covenant with all of nature (see Gen. 9:13-15). Dominion implies the responsibility to serve nature in what is essentially a stewardship relationship. God calls upon the Christian to exhibit dominion over nature without being destructive.

Unfortunately, God's command to "subdue" the earth (Gen. 1:28) has served as a sweeping rationalization for mindless exploitation of natural resources. Christians, of all people, should not be the destroyers. We should treat nature with an overwhelming respect.
MAX TORKELSEN

*What can I do to help preserve the national resources that God created for our use and management?*

# Fighting the Civilized War

*Then, because so many people were coming and going that they did not even have a chance to eat, he said to them, "Come with me by yourselves to a quiet place and get some rest." Mark 6:31, NIV.*

As long ago as the Civil War people were aware of it. Back then palpitations of the heart were so common among military troops that the condition became known as "soldier's heart."

During World War I a crippling anxiety developed among soldiers. Physicians referred to it as "shell shock" because they thought it to be caused by heavy artillery.

By the time World War II came along, the symptoms were called "battle fatigue." Then veterans of the Vietnam War experienced "post-traumatic stress disorder."

We now know that all of these illnesses had a single cause. The soldiers succumbed to a constant barrage of stressful combat episodes. They could find no rest, no renewal. And in this unending fight-or-flight environment, their reserve systems eventually collapsed.

But you're not in a war—or are you? Chances are you're involved in never-ending battles with job pressures, finances, and family problems. If you sometimes want to run away from it all, you're a casualty of the modern "civilized" war.

Alvin Toffler's book *Future Shock* describes this civilized war as "the distress both physical and psychological that arises from an overload of . . . adaptive systems and decision-making processes. Put more simply, [it] is the human response to overstimulation."

Overstimulation equals overload. It's estimated that we are subjected to 100 times more stressors than were our grandparents. Toffler insists that the civilized war exposes us to too much input in three areas:

1. *Sensory overload.* The human body responds to noise as it does to fear and anger. Even pleasant sounds at too high a volume can trigger a fight-or-flight response in us, and since World War II noise levels in the United States have increased 32-fold.

2. *Informational overload.* We live in the midst of an informational explosion, bombarding us with jangling telephones, daily newspapers, weekly magazines, home entertainment units, AM-FM radios, paperback books, monthly magazines, and home computers.

3. *Decisional overload.* Toffler suggests we are assaulted with a minimum of 560 advertising messages each day!

DeWitt S. Williams

*Lord, help me to tune out life's stressors and tune in to You.*

# An Emptiness
# That Will Never Be Filled

*Why are you downcast, O my soul? Why so disturbed within me? Put your hope in God, for I will yet praise him, my Savior and my God. Ps. 42:5, NIV.*

**M**ake her breathe, Peter! Make her breathe!"
My mind screamed the words to our obstetrician friend, but the delivery room was deadly silent. The child who moments before had been kicking in my womb was now cradled in his hands. So tiny; so fragile. He handed our daughter to me and my husband, and we held her as her heart slowed and finally stopped. Her lungs were too premature to take even one small breath.

I stared at the perfect features of my little girl, etching them forever in my mind. Although I felt the warmth go out of the doll-like body, I still could not give her up. I asked for a basin of water, and with the help of a friend washed her and wrapped her in a soft, white blanket. Then I rocked her gently.

We brought our other children in to see the sister who would never grow up to be their friend. When they had gone, my husband tenderly lifted her from my arms. "They're here for her. You have to let her go."

Of course I did, but it broke my heart.

I thought the tears would never stop. Then to add to the pain, an infection kept me in the hospital through the maze of following days and nights and the funeral. My homecoming, when it finally arrived, was not one of victory, but of desperation. Healing resulted from my physician husband's skilled hands and my sister-in-law's loving arms.

My mind cleared slowly, as if a fog were being burned off by the scent of the lilacs and the laughter of my children. Life returned to what would now be normal. But even after all these years, not a day passes that I don't think of my baby. There is an emptiness deep inside that will never be filled. Oh, how I long for her resurrection!

I wonder, as I think of my pain, how God's heart must break over the eternal loss of even one of His children. I have the feeling an emptiness deep inside Him will never be filled either!

KATHY KUZMA

*What event in your life makes you long for heaven?*

# The Dreaded Word: Alzheimer's

*Have mercy on me, O God, have mercy on me, for in you my soul takes refuge. I will take refuge in the shadow of your wings until the disaster has passed. Ps. 57:1, NIV.*

Alzheimer's—the word filled my mind with dread, fear, anger, and a chilling sense of hopelessness. The doctor was compassionate yet direct, knowing that my family needed to confront the reality as quickly as possible. Dad had given indications that things had changed—getting lost driving to familiar places, neglecting to finish a project, giving a puzzled glance when conversation didn't flow easily—situations that always came effortlessly for him before. The reality was that we were going to lose him, not in an immediate, physical way, but through a slow and sad deterioration of his mind. An odd sense of urgency came over me. I must live every precious moment I could with the man whom I could always find myself in a debate with, and who loved me dearly.

I questioned God's role in this. How did He fit into our inescapable tragedy? Where did miracles tie in with what we were facing? Why Dad? Tough questions to grapple with, and answers did not come—at least, not for a while.

Dad became carefree, happy, and oblivious to the tragedy, while our family began working through the emotions of shock, denial, and grief, then rapidly moved toward a sense of camaraderie and communication. We would have family councils to talk openly about our fears and together discover our talents and abilities to meet those challenges.

Slowly I began to see God's hand in our little world. He didn't cause Alzheimer's, but He did guide us to Emory University, where Mom and Dad were able to be part of a research team/support group. God didn't move mountains to cure the illness or restore Dad's vocabulary, but He did create opportunity for finding creative talents in our family and friends to meet the specific needs.

Where was God and why did it happen? I don't have all the answers, but I am at peace knowing that He gave us strength and comfort through the actions of family, friends, and the medical professionals who loved Dad. And really, it won't be long until Dad and I can debate once again—only this time it will be on things infinitely more fascinating.

CONNIE COBLE STARKEY

*Just as the rainbow follows the rain, smiles follow the pain. If you look for the blessings in the bad things, you'll find them. Let God be your refuge.*

# A Modern-Day Miracle

*This is the assurance we have in approaching God: that if we ask anything according to his will, he hears us. And if we know that he hears us—whatever we ask—we know that we have what we asked of him. 1 John 5:14, 15, NIV.*

In the early 1970s I was working on the morning shift as a nurse at the orthopedic surgery unit at Loma Linda University Medical Center.

Many of the patients there were older women who had broken their hips. After menopause a woman's bones demineralize and weaken. Since the hip is a major weight-bearing joint, often their hips would break and they would fall, rather than falling first and breaking their hips from the blow. The treatment, then, rather than months in a plaster cast, was surgery in which a metal nail would be used to stabilize the fracture.

This story is about one such woman. The relationship she had with her grown sons caught everyone's attention. They were loving and kind. One or both would come every day to sit with her while she ate and to help her.

Her wound, however, instead of healing, became infected. Despite our best efforts, she got worse and worse.

My heart ached for her. I wanted to help her, so I turned to God. I felt so unworthy to ask for a miracle healing. While I had no doubt in my mind that God *could* heal her, *would* He? I knew it had to be her faith, as well as mine, so I went to her bedside and asked her if she believed in God. "Oh, yes," she said, so I asked God to heal her, if it was His will, and then we thanked Him for answering our prayer.

The next day I hesitantly went into her room. She looked up at me and smiled one of the most beautiful smiles I had ever seen. I noticed her cheeks were rosy! Trembling, I removed the dressing from her hip wound. I could not believe my eyes. It looked as if two full weeks of healing had taken place overnight. We praised God. She fully recovered and went home to her family.

I believe God healed her to help her, but also so that this story could be told to strengthen my faith and that of others.

JANENE JENKINS

*God is a God of miracles. Approach Him with the words of Psalm 150: "Praise the Lord! Praise God in His sanctuary; praise Him in His mighty firmament! Praise Him for His mighty acts; praise Him according to His excellent greatness!" (NKJV).*

# 23 Traits of a Strong, Healthy Family

*Unless the Lord builds the house, its builders labor in vain. Ps. 127:1, NIV.*

Researchers have found that the majority of strong, healthy families have the following traits in common:

1. **Commitment:** Put God and your family first, and commit to helping each other become everything God designed you to be.

2. **Appreciation and affirmation:** Give positive attention and affirm each other, letting each family member know they're special. Strong families focus on the strengths of each other, not the faults.

3. **Time together:** Healthy families enjoy being together. Work together, play together, and enjoy leisure times together. Family members may be busy, but they don't let jobs, school, or personal hobbies steal family time.

4. **Communication:** To understand each other a family has to be willing to invest the time necessary to share their feelings and opinions. Each day

you are a new person. Without sharing those experiences with each other, family members can soon become strangers.

5. **Religion:** Sharing a religious faith and having similar religious values and standards is extremely important. Worshipping together is a bonding experience. But most important is a commitment to God, the foundation of the family.

6. **Play and a sense of humor:** Happy families have fun together; they play together; they laugh together. Having a sense of humor during troublesome moments is like pouring oil on restless water. It defuses the tension and has an immediate calming effect.

7. **Sharing responsibilities and roles:** If family members will do whatever is necessary to meet each other's needs, even if the task doesn't happen to be on their priority list, everyone is happier. Be flexible and responsible.

8. **Common interests and goals:** The more a family has in common, the more its members tend to do together. Having similar interests and getting behind common goals gives the family something to look forward to, to plan, and to experience together.

9. **Service to others:** Just as a pond grows stagnant if it has no outlet, so does a family. Reaching out and helping others bonds families together.

10. **Admitting to and seeking help with problems:** Healthy families aren't problem-free; they just admit to problems and get the help they need to solve them!

KAY KUZMA

*How does your family measure up? For a little bit of heaven on earth, make God the foundation of your family and add these 10 essential traits.* 52

# Battling Busyness

*Remember the Sabbath day by keeping it holy. Ex. 20:8, NIV.*

**D**o you sometimes feel you're losing the battle with busyness? Take advantage of God's winning weapon: the Sabbath.

The fourth commandment says: "Six days you shall labor and do all your work, but the seventh day is a Sabbath to the Lord your God. On it you shall not do any work" (Ex. 20:9, 10, NIV).

During the six days of labor each week you may feel you're coming apart at the seams. But one day each week you receive permission—yes, are commanded—to come apart in a different way.

• Come apart from the noise of alarm clocks, machinery, traffic, telephones.

• Come apart from the information-bearers: newspaper, radio, TV, fax machines, and computers.

• Come apart from the rush: schedules, Day-Timers, freeways, airports, taxis, watches.

• Come apart from the clamoring for decisions: those endless committee meetings and conference calls.

• Come apart from the busyness of life—and rest in the assurance of God's love, His salvation, and the value that He places on *you*—not on what you do.

The Sabbath commandment is more for us today than for any people in human history. Of the Sabbath, Abraham Joshua Heschel writes: "There is a realm of time where the goal is not to have but to be, not to own but to give, not to control but to share, not to subdue but to be in accord. Life goes wrong when the control of space, the acquisition of things of space, becomes our sole concern."

During the week our very self-image becomes embroiled in our busyness. The Sabbath, however, rests on a revolutionary concept: we have value beyond what we produce. God values us just for being us, for being His children. That's what the Sabbath is all about.

As Tilden Edwards notes: "Stopping work tests our trust: will the world and I fall apart if I stop making things happen for a while?"

The busyness of modern life cripples our stamina, wounds our self-image, shatters our joy. But the Sabbath celebrates the wonder of being totally alive.

DeWitt S. Williams

*Lord, thank You for the Sabbath. How wonderful it is that You have created that day for us so we can rest from the busyness of life.*

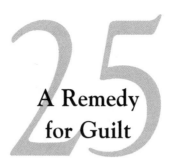

# A Remedy
# for Guilt

*All that the Father gives Me shall come to Me; and the one who comes to Me I will certainly not cast out. John 6:37, NASB.*

The headline virtually screamed the word "GUILTY." The photo beneath it could break a heart. It showed a mother and father bidding farewell to their beloved 18-year-old daughter before guards led her away to serve the next 10 years or more in prison for the alleged murder of her newly born infant.

The love and pain mingled in their faces strikes to the heart of anyone who has loved a child—to the heart of anyone who has loved anyone. What true parents have not dreamed dreams and hoped hopes for their children? What parents have not labored and sacrificed to help these hopes come true? College . . . music lessons . . . ball games . . .

Such a scene reminds one that for all of us, when called to stand before God, the righteous Judge, and answer for our lives, the verdict will be guilty! The Bible tells us that *"all* have sinned" (Rom. 3:23).

But in our hurting love for a straying or troubled child another picture comes to mind—a picture of God, our Father, who emptied all heaven on our behalf and spent His most cherished possession to redeem us. God did something for us that the young girl's parents were unable to do for her. Isaiah 53:5-9 tells how He took our punishment! "But he was pierced for our transgressions, he was crushed for our iniquities. . . . We all, like sheep, have gone astray, each of us has turned to his own way; and the Lord has laid on him the iniquity of us all" (NIV).

Our way of dealing with another's guilt (or supposed guilt) is to throw stones and to separate the troubled person from the very sources and community that might render aid. Someone has referred to it as "shooting our wounded."

The Lord does not let the guilty go free, but He does offer a solution—a solution that, were it practiced among us as family, friends, community, and church, would restore many a troubled, hurting soul. With heart and arms wide open, He pleads, "Come unto me" (Matt. 11:28). His promise is that He will not cast out any who do so (see John 6:37).

LOIS (RITTENHOUSE) PECCE

*Is there someone who needs your example of God's love and acceptance?*

# Not All Calories Are Equal

*When you sit to dine with a ruler, note well what is before you, and put a knife to your throat if you are given to gluttony. Do not crave his delicacies for that food is deceptive. Prov. 23:1-3, NIV.*

You can't just cut your calories and expect to lose weight. Here's why: By nature, your body is highly efficient in storing fat calories. It uses only about 3 percent of the fat calories you eat to digest, transport, and deposit fat into your body's fat storage areas. That means you must exercise the vast majority out of the body if you don't want to gain weight.

In contrast, your body metabolizes protein calories and excretes the by-products rapidly. You can have problems with excess protein, of course, because it stresses your liver and kidneys by forcing them to work overtime. But excess protein doesn't usually add to obesity. You have no efficient metabolic pathway in your body by which you can turn protein into fat for storage.

Calories from carbohydrates also rarely get stored as fat, because the metabolic pathways that your body uses to convert extra carbohydrates into fat and then store them demand that you burn a lot of calories to do the job. It take 24 percent of the calories in carbohydrates to do this—a highly inefficient use of the energy in the carbohydrates.

In studies in which researchers put radioactive carbohydrate markers in food, they learned that the body converted and stored less than 1 percent of the carbohydrate load as fat. Even when people ate carbohydrates excessively, they generally burned them up in "wasteful" metabolic processes that tended to increase the body's metabolic rate, not reduce it—as happens in calorie-restricted diets.

Another way to put this is that one gram of fat contains nine calories, while one gram of protein or carbohydrates has only four calories.

The moral of the story is: avoid fat calories—they stick to your bones!

There's an interesting bit of advice in Proverbs 23:3 about overeating. It says don't crave a ruler's delicacies, because that food is deceptive. How true! Most rich food is filled with fat calories that may be tough to get rid of.

Sin is deceptive, too. It may look and taste good, but the consequences of indulging may be even harder to get rid of than fat calories.

JAN W. KUZMA AND CECIL MURPHEY

*Watch your moral diet, "for the wages of sin is death" (Rom. 6:23).*

# I Chose How
# I Wanted to Feel

*The wrong desires that come into your life aren't anything new and different. . . . And no temptation is irresistible. You can trust God to keep the temptation from becoming so strong that you can't stand up against it, . . . He will show you how to escape temptation's power. 1 Cor. 10:13, TLB.*

**A**s executive director of a Christian ministry made up of thousands of members who take care of one another's medical bills, you would think I would have known better. I was 45 percent overweight, was on three heart medications, was taking pain medication for arthritis, had lower back pain, had reoccurring diverticulosis, was listless, and had shortness of breath. I had one criteria for eating, and that was "How does it taste?"

Finally I admitted that I was powerless in my own strength to change and desperately needed God's help. An acquaintance introduced me to some basic nutritional information that led me to eat only fruits and vegetables for 10 days so as to cleanse my body. My cravings totally changed in that time. Next I made a conscious choice between how I wanted to feel and how I wanted things to taste. Choosing how I wanted to feel, I later discovered new tastes with even greater fulfillment than the old.

Then a friend gave me *Counsels on Diet and Foods*. I found the book instructive and extremely advanced. I began to see my problem as one of lust of the flesh. I was enslaved to the first inch of my tongue.

Now, 17 months later, I am off all pain and heart medication, am 80 pounds lighter, and have more energy than any time since my college days (I am closer to 60 than 50). Last fall my son and I enjoyed hiking six to eight miles a day. I found myself praising the Lord for a new life and outlook.

Can you see the parallels? After we come to a point where we admit that we are powerless against sin, we turn to a gracious Lord who is ready, willing, and able to change us from the inside out. We repent, enjoy His cleansing, and launch a life based on choices pleasing to Him and best for us. He rewards us by giving us fulfillment and blessings. Then He brings people into our paths to touch us and help us on our way, while also leading us to those we can help.

God is the giver of new life. How can we not adore Him?

E. JOHN REINHOLD

*Are you choosing how you want things to taste over how you want to feel? Give the 10-day fruit and vegetable diet a chance to reeducate your taste to the delights of God's original diet.*

# 28 Cherish Your Vitality

*Then because so many people were coming and going that they did not even have a chance to eat, he said to them, "Come with me by yourselves to a quiet place and get some rest." So they went away by themselves . . . to a solitary place. Mark 6:30-32, NIV.*

Jesus knew His personal ministry on earth wouldn't last long, and one of His main objectives was to train His disciples to carry on when He was gone. Therefore, it was important to use every opportunity for them to gain the instruction and experience they would need. It was an intense course of study.

Even at the end of each day their work was not finished. If they were to take time out, many of the needy people would not receive the help they needed. So it was only natural that they would try to work continuously lest they neglect any opportunity. But even so, the Master arranged for a period of relaxation and rejuvenation. He placed a higher priority on the need for preserving vitality and efficiency than on continuously responding to whatever cried for their attention.

It is clear that working beyond one's capabilities,

even in a worthy enterprise, carries the risk of defeat. Take the case of Margery, a 34-year-old schoolteacher and mother of three, who was beginning to suffer from migraine headaches. Typical of most persons who suffer from migraine, she was a highly organized and efficient mother, homemaker, and teacher. She did all this, however, by sheer determination and at the price of not having time to consider the beauties and blessings that surrounded her. Margery felt personally responsible for her pupils' progress and her family's comfort and welfare. But she was not taking time to replenish the energy she was consuming.

What would remedy the headaches? Should she quit? Not necessarily. Margery needed to reconsider her personal limitations and adopt a new lifestyle in which she shared her responsibilities with others. She could petition the school board to provide a volunteer aid for her classroom and could counsel with her husband and children to see how she could be relieved of some routine home duties. Most of all, she needed time to be by herself and think, pray, and relax.

HAROLD SHRYOCK

*Just as Jesus summoned His disciples apart to replenish their energy, He is calling you. What changes do you need to make in your life so you can do as He urges?*

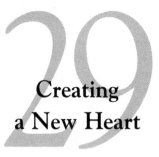

# Creating
# a New Heart

*Cleanse me with hyssop, and I will be clean; wash me, and I will be whiter than snow. . . . Create in me a pure heart, O God, and renew a steadfast spirit within me.* Ps. 51:7-10, NIV.

**T**wice I had gone to the emergency room to treat a pulse rate of more than 160 beats per minute that had lasted several hours each time. Each time it took intravenous medications to slow the too-rapid rate. Treating my problem required careful monitoring and other specific medications and emergency equipment. The cardiologist said it could be cured. The treatment was a procedure called ablation.

In just a few days my doctor had me scheduled for the ablation. I checked in at the hospital early in the morning. Two physicians, a nurse, and a technician attended me.

They threaded four electrodes into the large vein of my groin that carries blood to the right atrium of my heart. One electrode went into my jugular vein and on into my right atrium. One cardiologist manipulated the five electrodes while the other cardiologist, with the aid of a computer, monitored my heart's reaction as the electrodes searched the inner surface of the heart chamber for the misfiring circuit of my heart. Once the team located the culprit, the technician with a second computer applied heat to burn out unwanted tissue.

As the technician applied the heat, I felt a very warm sensation in the area I thought my heart occupied. The warm heart made me feel good all over. The team did the burnout of unwanted cardiac tissue two more times. Each time I savored the warm glow. I wanted to keep that wonderful warm feeling forever. In five and a half hours they had completed the procedure, and the cardiologist gave me the good news. I would not need a pacemaker.

What about the sin in my heart? To remove it will not need two physicians, one nurse, a technician, and two computers with monitors and five electrodes. *Only Jesus.* He is the creator of clean hearts—instantly, as soon as you invite Him in.

Jesus doesn't take five and a half hours, nor is scheduling necessary. Simply invite Him in. The warm glow of His presence is a warmth that never goes away.

ELIZABETH STERNDALE

*O God, create in me a clean heart. May I feel the healing presence of Your Spirit! May Jesus' love fill my soul this day and every day. Amen.*

# Either Burn Out or Delegate

*"Why do you alone sit as judge, while all these people stand around you from morning till evening?" . . . "What you are doing is not good. You and these people who come to you will only wear yourselves out. The work is too heavy for you. . . . Select capable men . . . and appoint them as officials." Ex. 18:14-21, NIV.*

**D**uring the time that Moses was involved in the liberation of the Israelites from Egypt, he had left his wife and two sons with Jethro, his father-in-law. When Jethro heard that the Israelites were migrating near to where he lived, he took Zipporah and their boys back to Moses.

Soon Jethro noticed a problem. Moses didn't have any time for them—or for himself, for that matter. So Jethro spoke up and basically said that even though Moses was God's appointed leader of the children of Israel, that didn't mean he had to do everything himself. Read this fascinating story for yourself in Exodus 18.

For the first 40 years of his life Moses had been trained in the court of Egypt in matters of government and administration, so he had great ability in dealing with people. Now he had a divine mandate to educate and train God's people in loyalty to their

Creator. A conscientious person, Moses felt a great sense of responsibility and urgency for those under his charge.

Jethro understood that Moses was unselfishly doing his best to fulfill his God-given commission. But he also recognized that Moses was in danger of burnout. Israel's leader was exerting himself in a most worthy cause, but that did not justify his being presumptuous in expecting the Lord's continued blessing.

So Jethro said to Moses, "Listen now to me and I will give you some advice, and may God be with you" (Ex. 18:19, NIV). He then outlined an administrative structure in which Moses would continue to be the people's representative to God, and God's representative to the people, but would also train others to administer groups of thousands, hundreds, fifties, and tens. "That will make your load lighter, because they will share it with you" (verse 22).

Then he said, "If you do this and God so commands, you will be able to stand the strain, and all these people will go home satisfied" (verse 23). And Moses too could go home at a decent time to his wife and children, who also needed him!

HAROLD SHRYOCK

*Are you trying to do more than your share? Ask the Holy Spirit and your family how you could cut down before you burn out.*

# 31

# Was I Going to Die?

*Peace I leave with you; my peace I give you. I do not give to you as the world gives. Do not let your hearts be troubled and do not be afraid. John 14:27, NIV.*

I was scared. Was I going to die? Would my boys be motherless? And would my husband love me less if I had to have a mastectomy?

I had just received news of a mass in my left breast. It was our twenty-first wedding anniversary. A hushed reserve hung over us as we ate our special dinner together, and later, as we sat in our hotel room, we talked about what the future might hold.

By Friday, without our anniversary celebration to think about, the depressing "what if" feelings crept in. I prayed constantly, and forced myself to sing and be happy. But the next day in church, thoughts of possible death and despair overwhelmed me, and I broke down. The statistics kept ringing in my ears. After lung cancer, breast cancer is the leading cancer killer of U.S. women.

On Sunday we both went to see the surgeon, and we were encouraged. He felt that it was possibly a fibrocystic nodule. Saying that he wanted to see me in two months, he put me on a strict diet and increased exercise. According to research findings, an extra 15 pounds increases the risk of breast cancer by 37 percent, and with an extra 20 pounds the risk rises to 52 percent. That means that a 10-pound difference may be significant when it comes to lowering your cancer risk. And according to Dr. Noreen Azid, of the Lee Moffit Cancer Center in Tampa, Florida, of all the decades of life you should lose that extra weight, it's the third one.

The weeks passed, and I had lost 12 pounds. Allan went with me to see the doctor. Following an ultrasound and mammogram, the doctor reported: "There is no mass." After comparing the reports and seeing the mammogram, we sighed in relief and sent a prayer heavenward in thanksgiving.

From that experience we learned how precious is our health, and how its threatened loss can suddenly and markedly rearrange our priorities. Continually I resolve to appreciate each day the Lord gives and to be glad and rejoice in it.

JILL KENNEDY

*What should you do today, in case there is no tomorrow?*

# Igniting Potential

*" 'If you can'?" said Jesus. "Everything is possible for him who believes." Mark 9:23, NIV.*

Leslie Lemke has the ability to reproduce on the piano anything he hears. But the incredible thing is that not only is Leslie blind, but he's also crippled with cerebral palsy and severely disabled mentally! Here's his story:

Leslie was born prematurely and abandoned as hopelessly disabled. He had already lost his sight when May Lemke, a 52-year-old nurse, decided to quit her job to raise the pathetic 6-month-old child everyone thought was hopeless. Everyone, that is, except May. As the days of her patient, loving care stretched into years, she saw few signs of improvement.

But May didn't give up. She knew God had given Leslie a gift, and she prayed she would have the wisdom to help him find it.

May carried him everywhere until he was too heavy to lift. Then she stood him beside the backyard fence, hoping he would hang on and stand by himself, but he just crumpled into a heap. Eventually he did stand, and then walked. But he still didn't talk.

The boy did one thing, however, that seemed out of the ordinary. Whenever he touched a piece of taut string or wire, he would pick at it with his fingers. The day May found him strumming rhythmically on the bedsprings she suspected Leslie might be musical. So she and her husband bought a used piano and put it in Leslie's bedroom.

Then came the task of teaching him to play. She had him listen to classical music by the hour. Then she placed his fingers on the keys and explained the sounds he heard. And finally, after years of "practice," he began picking out simple tunes.

Early one morning, when Leslie was 16, May woke up to a flawless performance of Tchaikovsky's Piano Concerto No. 1. She rushed into Leslie's room and found him sitting at his piano reproducing perfectly the music he had grown to love. Three years later he said his first word.

It's an incredible story, isn't it? But every person has God-given possibilities, if we will just look for them in ourselves and in others!

KAY KUZMA

*Dear Lord, help me to see possibilities in myself and others. Amen.*

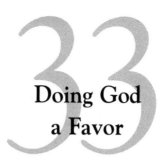

# Doing God
a Favor

*Fathers, do not provoke your children to anger, but bring them up in the discipline and instruction of the Lord. Eph. 6:4, RSV.*

The following fact is both good news and bad news! Almost everything our children will come to believe about God will be powerfully shaped by what they see in their parents. And most of a child's feelings about God will be formed when parents are fulfilling what some regard as our most Godlike responsibility: teaching them to obey.

Unfortunately, we as parents don't get any children to practice on. We have to make all our parenting mistakes, all our test runs and learning labs, on real children—even as our parents learned so much by watching what happened to us when they made some blunders.

Quite likely the apostle Paul had this in mind when he cautioned fathers about making their children angry. But let's face it—it's almost a given that when fatherly authority comes head-to-head against the high energy and freewheeling curiosity of youth, someone's going to get angry. Dad has to say no long before the children can understand why—which doesn't prevent a three-foot-tall challenge to adult dignity from insisting "Why?" At this point, anger is often just a blink away.

We face no more delicate task than that of helping human beings, who sense that they are moral agents, learn to live within the boundaries of reality. When parents believe that they can accomplish this by their power, by their ability to "make them obey" through the threat of pain or physical force, they not only make their children angry, but also give God a black eye.

Though we use big Latin words such a "omnipotent" and draw images from notions of royalty such as "King of kings" to celebrate God's great dignity, our God simply does not stoop to the use of power and force to win the free, thoughtful loyalty of His friends—His created beings! Rather, He helps us understand the built-in benefits of choosing to live by His principles. And who can be angry about that?

RICHARD WINN

*Are you giving God a black eye by the way you treat your children and others?*

# The Health Benefits of Generosity

*Command them to do good, to be rich in good deeds, and to be generous and willing to share. In this way they will lay up treasure for themselves as a firm foundation for the coming age, so that they may take hold of the life that is truly life. 1 Tim. 6:18, 19, NIV.*

When John D. Rockefeller was in his 50s he was broken in health and ready to die as the richest man in the United States. It was said that the veins in his arms were as hard as lead pipes. He was a driven man—driven to satisfy his lust for material wealth—and had used every possible means available to him to make money and destroy his competitors.

As Rockefeller faced death he began to see himself for the greedy fool he really was, and to fear his encounter with God. Maybe if he used his money to meet the needs of others, he thought, God would forgive him for the way he had acquired his wealth.

He resolved to become kind and benevolent, and began giving away millions. Instead of dying, he steadily improved in health. He was also far happier in his money-giving days than he had been in his money-making days. When he died at the ripe old age of 97, it was said that the veins in his arms were as soft as a baby's.

Long before Rockefeller, the Bible illustrated the health principle of generosity with the story of two rich farmers.

The farmer in Luke 12:16-21 had a problem. His harvest was so bountiful his barns weren't large enough to store it. In a purely selfish but very logical decision, the man ordered larger grain elevators built, and then stretched out in his recliner and gloated over how lavishly he had provided for himself for years to come so he could take it easy, eat, drink, and be merry. Jesus called him a fool, because that night the man died and someone else inherited his wealth.

The second was Boaz. In contrast, Boaz allowed the poor to glean in his fields. He was particularly generous with a foreign-born widow, Ruth, and later married her. Because of his generosity he became the great-grandfather of King David and a forerunner of the Saviour Himself (Ruth 2-4).

When you're tempted to accumulate things for yourself, remember the scriptural health principle: "It is more blessed to give than to receive" (Acts 20:35).

JEFFREY K. WILSON

*What more could you do to practice the health principle of generosity?*

# 35

# Green Garden Gold

*Now the Lord God had planted a garden in the east, in Eden; and there he put the man he had formed. And the Lord God made all kinds of trees grow out of the ground—trees that were pleasing to the eye and good for food. Gen. 2:8, 9, NIV.*

Growing a garden is good for your health.

It may sound like work, but pruning some trees and sowing some seeds out in the fresh air might be just what you need to lower stress in your life, clear your mind of worries, and help you get the exercise you need to feel better. In fact, just viewing beautiful landscapes can alter blood pressure, heart rate, and muscle tension!

Joel Flagler, an agricultural agent at Rutgers University, says more people garden than any other leisure activity because "it's a wonderful way to counteract stress, refresh yourself, and become more productive."

Studies on people in prisons and mental hospitals report that working with plants releases nurturing instincts and makes them feel useful and renewed. "Role reversals occur when patients who require constant care become caregivers for living things," says Flagler. It makes them feel better about themselves.

But a garden offers more health benefits than just stress-reduction. If you eat fruits and vegetables grown in good soil, without pesticides, you have the best possible chance of getting all the vitamins and minerals your body needs.

For example, low trace mineral levels have been correlated with such problems as allergies, diabetes mellitus, hypertension, and arthritis. We get such minerals primarily from our food. In an attempt to determine how commercially grown food compared with homegrown or organically grown food, it was found that in most instances the organic food won, with 240 percent more iron, 120 percent more manganese, and 100 percent more zinc than commercial foods.

All these health benefits from gardening are enough to keep me pruning and planting. And as I look at my Goldcot apricots and rose-blushed Gala apples, and bite into that incredibly sweet, juicy Belle of Georgia peach, I have no doubt in my mind that it was all worth it.

I think God knew what He was doing when He planted a garden for Adam and Eve. It doesn't say He spoke it into being—it says *He planted it!* For the sake of your health, maybe it's time you followed your Creator's example!

JAN W. KUZMA

*Think about what you could plant this season. Maybe a patio tomato, a cucumber vine, and some radish seeds, and enjoy God's green garden gold.*

# Bicycle Bob
## and His Wife Theresa

*Then He who sat on the throne said, "Behold, I make all things new." And He said to me, "Write, for these words are true and faithful." Rev. 21:5, NKJV.*

When Bob Anderson was 66 he retired as a building contractor because of debilitating arthritis in his lower back. "I could hardly make it out to the mailbox," Bob said, "so I started driving my old car the 200 feet to get the mail. I had no energy. I was 60 pounds overwheight, smoked three packs of cigarettes a day, and was always short of breath."

His wife's health wasn't much better. Theresa suffered from high blood pressure and diabetes and was overweight and extremely depressed.

Then Dr. Hans Diehl came to their town of Creston, British Columbia, with a Live With All Your Heart Seminar. Its message was simple: "Our diets are killing us. Our excesses in meat, rich dairy products, sugar, alcohol, salt, and tobacco must go, or we'll eat and drink ourselves into early graves."

The results of their HeartScreen health evaluation jolted the Andersons into action. Their blood pressure, cholesterol, and blood sugar were all too high. When they realized their rich diet and sedentary lifestyle were contributing to their heart disease, diabetes, hypertension, and osteoarthritis, they dumped their vodka down the sink and filled three garbage bags with the "junk" food they cleaned out of their refrigerator. They burned Bob's cigarettes (a 35-year-long habit) in their fireplace, and started walking. First just one block, then two, three, five—and more.

They say God can make crooked things straight, and that happened to Bob. By the sixth month his back pain disappeared; he stood straight and walked without a limp. Their blood pressure, cholesterol, and blood sugar levels returned to normal. Both took up bicycling and shed 50 pounds, and three years later, at age 69, Bob cycled 3,210 miles from Creston to Ottawa, Ontario, in 60 days.

Theresa says, "No more are we simply enduring retirement. We are living our lives to the hilt! We both have bicycles and love life on the road. And as our physical health improves, we are growing spiritually. We've been born again and are active in our church. Now we have a purpose and sense of direction in our lives."

AILEEN LUDINGTON

*If you don't want to just endure retirement, the time to do something about your lifestyle is now. Determine what must change in your life, and make a commitment to God that you will start your new life today.*

# Fill Your Mouth With Laughter

*He will yet fill your mouth with laughing, and your lips with rejoicing. Job 8:21, NKJV.*

Laughter may indeed be the best medicine after all. In his *Anatomy of an Illness*, published in 1979, Norman Cousins recounts how 10 minutes of solid belly laughter would give him two hours of pain-free sleep. Laughter stimulates heart and blood circulation and promotes respiration. It produces deep relaxation, thereby breaking up our tension.

Just putting on a happy face can be rewarding. Working in a high-rise for senior citizens for several years, I made what I thought at the time was the profound discovery that if I smiled—*whether I felt like it or not*—I would feel better. I knew I couldn't go in to those old people looking like a grump, so I would paste on a smile, and soon I was actually smiling. In an article published in the Orlando *Sentinel*, Ronald S. Miller states that "if we just assume facial expressions of happiness, we can increase blood flow to the brain and stimulate release of favorable neurotransmitters." So when I smile I am releasing neurotransmitters and giving others—and myself—a better day in the process!

Years ago I had a ministry with parents who had lost children. At the risk of sounding like a heretic, I asked them to keep a good joke book beside the Bible. I explained that there would be days when even the Bible might need to be supplemented with a good laugh that could, at least momentarily, lift the incredible weight of pain and loss. My personal daily shot in the funny bone is Lynn Johnston's *For Better or for Worse*. God bless her for her painkiller insight on family life.

One more bit of advice: don't stick around negative people. These are what one writer calls "energy suckers." Do yourself a huge favor and find someone positive and funny and enjoy life.

God wants us to laugh and enjoy the full range of positive emotions He created. Otherwise, He wouldn't have promised to "fill your mouth with laughter and your lips with rejoicing"!

So let's rattle those funny bones today and praise our heavenly Father for the wonderful gift of laughter.

PAT NORDMAN

*If 10 minutes of laughter helped Norman Cousins sleep pain-free for two hours, what might it do for your health?*

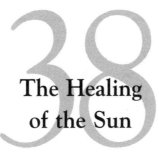

# The Healing
of the Sun

*For you who revere my name, the sun of righteousness will
rise with healing in its wings. And you will go out and leap like
calves released from the stall. Mal. 4:2, NIV.*

The ship arrived at Antarctica December 24,
1928. Richard Byrd and his crew of 41 unloaded
supplies for Little America—the place they would
stay for the next 14 months. When they arrived, the
sun shone for 24 hours. As the men worked, they
knew time only by checking their watches.

Then the length of days began to decrease, and
in April they lost the sun. They lived in buildings
connected by underground tunnels for five months.
During this time the morale of the men deteriorated
significantly. Then on August 20, 1929, the sun returned. Norman Vaughn writes in his autobiography
*With Byrd at the Bottom of the World:* "How can I explain the joyousness of the first few days of sunlight?
We felt like prisoners who had received commuta-
tion of our sentences. A brightness appeared on our
faces. We walked faster and moved with an energy
we had long forgotten."

Do you take the sun for granted? It has incredible health-giving properties such as killing germs, helping our bodies manufacture vitamin D, and improving the function of our pituitary, hypothalamus, and pineal glands. Plus, it's essential for growing our food. The simple fact is, we can't function without the sun. Nor can we function without the Sun of righteousness.

I can just imagine Admiral Byrd's party coming out of their underground homes, seeing the light of the sun, and kicking up their heels with joy, can't you? This same joy can be yours each morning as you welcome God's new day, and as you invite the Sun of righteousness into your life. Experience the reality of the promise in Malachi: "For you who revere my name, the sun of righteousness will rise with healing in its wings. And you will go out and leap like calves released from the stall."

Light is the starting place of life. Perhaps that's why the biblical account of Creation begins this way: "In the beginning . . . God said, 'Let there be light,' and there was light. God saw that the light was good" (Gen. 1:1-4, NIV).

JAN W. KUZMA AND CECIL MURPHEY

*Spend some time today in the light God created for you to enjoy.*

# A Contented Mind

*And now, my friends, all that is true, all that is noble, all that is just and pure, all that is lovable and gracious, whatever is excellent and admirable—fill all your thoughts with these things. Phil. 4:8, NEB.*

While working as an Army physician, I noticed that near the end of the year many of the wives, especially those of servicemen on extended duty away from home, would come to the dispensary looking for tranquilizers.

However, one woman, a nurse, always had a smile on her face and a bubbly personality. Since this was quite unusual, I asked how she could keep such a sunny disposition while everyone around her was so nervous and depressed. Here was her response:

"Frequently people share gossip and other negative information about what is going on around the base. But when someone comes to my house, I invite them to have a seat while I continue working and listen to their chatter. But if they begin talking about who is having problems, whose children are getting into trouble, or whose husband or wife is unfaithful, I stop them and say, 'I have enough problems of my own, so I don't need to hear about others. If you want to talk happy, you are free to stay, but if you want to talk negative, you will have to leave.'

"As you can expect," she said laughingly, "I don't have many close friends, but those I have are positive.

"The second thing I do is keep my mind fresh and alive. Whenever I read about something in the news or the papers that I don't understand, I run to the library and ask the librarian if she can help me find books that I can understand to explain the problem area, so I always keep my mind filled with new information and positive thoughts. That's why I don't need medicine to keep me happy."

Two points that will help you keep a contented mind:

1. Avoid negative input—from anyone.
2. Keep improving your mind.

Paul said the same thing in our text for today. The secret to the successful Christian life lies not so much in what we do as in what we choose to let into our minds. Positive, kind, excellent, admirable, and praiseworthy thoughts breed the same kind of mind in us as was in Christ Jesus.

RICHARD NEIL

*What will you fill your mind with today?*

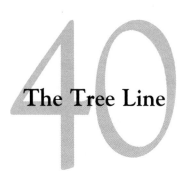

# The Tree Line

*Before his downfall a man's heart is proud, but humility comes before honor. Prov. 18:12, NIV.*

I've discovered in my years of exercising that a battle rages within my body—a contest between strength and flexibility, two goals that almost seem opposed to each other. I want to be strong, so I usually concentrate on strengthening activities (lifting weights, jogging, push-ups, etc.), which leave my muscles tight and rigid. But I know that I need to stay limber as well. If I neglect my stretching routine, I could easily pull a tight muscle at the wrong time.

As I hike the majestic peaks of the Sierra Nevadas, I'm reminded of the importance of flexibility. As the elevation of the mountain increases, trees begin to disappear, until at about 10,000 feet they cease to grow at all. This transition point is called the tree line. Near the tree line you often see a few twisted and misshapen trees, permanently bent by the relentless winds. Above the tree line even the mighty oak cannot survive the punishing winds and poor soil. At high altitude the barren and rocky terrain seems almost devoid of life. Almost—but not quite.

Look down low, and you will see the soft and supple willow clinging to the rocks, flourishing to a height of no more than six inches. While the mighty winds will crack and break the beefy oak at the craggy peaks, the lowly willow bends, and the wind passes on through.

It is as if God has placed before us a great visual lesson to remind us that the lofty heights of human existence are no place for the proud and haughty. Here only the lowly and humble will survive. God certainly does not discourage ambition and aspiration. Joseph and Daniel both showed great wisdom in the high-pressure, high-profile arena of world politics. But we dare not walk those heights alone, or like the mighty oak, we will be swept off the mountain.

So in my training routine I aim to be as strong as an oak but as supple as a willow. In this way I may also learn to stand for principle against the raging winds of temptation, but yield to my heavenly Father's will in modesty and humility.

LARRY RICHARDSON

*Lord, may I stand for principle and be modest and humble as I scale the heights of possibility within Your will. Amen.*

# Keeping Track
## of the Enemy

*Take heed, watch and pray; for you do not know when the time is. . . . And what I say to you, I say to all: Watch!* Mark 13:33-37, NKJV.

Have you ever wondered how Elijah could have become so disheartened and discouraged after the tremendous victory God gave him on Mount Carmel (1 Kings 18, 19)? After all, it was the same man ravens had already sustained miraculously in the wilderness! Yet in his fatigued, worn-out state Elijah's faith and confidence in God failed him. Suddenly terribly afraid, he ran for his life.

We, like Elijah, find ourselves in a contest between good and evil. It is a struggle just as fierce as the one on Mount Carmel, but it plays out in our lives daily.

Let's take a moment to look at the impact fatigue has on modern-day soldiers serving in artillery fire direction centers. Part of their job is to plot the location of artillery targets as requested by forward observers, and to update their situation maps continually.

Studies indicate that when a team has rested, it

performs very well. However, when tired, it ceases to keep up the situation map. As a result, its members lose grasp of their position in relationship to friendly and enemy units, and consequently often do not know what they are firing at!

We are like those soldiers too! When we are tired, our vigilance wanes. Our ability to set priorities and focus attention on the tasks at hand vanishes. The events and crises of life drive us, instead of the other way around. Yet we are unaware that anything has affected our performance!

Our Christian life suffers in exactly the same way. Fatigue lessens our spiritual vigilance. We're more likely to have lapses of attention, and it is at these weak moments that the enemy chooses to make his moves. During this state we also easily lose sight of the enemy, thus totally missing him and his maneuvers against us.

Do you consider fatigue a normal part of your life? Remember, fatigue profoundly affects your performance at home, at work, and for the Lord. It was not until Elijah had rested that his faith and confidence in God returned.

FRED HARDINGE

*Lord, help me to choose to get seven or eight hours of sleep each night so that I can remain a vigilant, watchful soldier for You!*

# God's Bonding
# Delight for Marriage

*Now Adam knew Eve his wife; and she conceived, and bare Cain. Gen. 4:1.*

While some more modern translations of the Bible may be more technically accurate, the King James Version portrays the story of Eve and Adam's marital union most sensitively and poetically. It takes sexual union out of the purely physical realm and gives it a dimension of wholeness.

When we say we "know" someone, as we use the term in daily speech, we mean that the person is more than an acquaintance. We feel that we have a relationship that includes respect, understanding, good feelings about, favorable regard for, and an interest in the other's activities and his or her thinking. Knowing someone well takes time, interest, and motivation.

When the King James translators used the word "know" to refer to the sexual experience of the first pair, they were saying something extremely profound. In order for sex to be the bonding delight God intended it to be, marital partners really need to "know" each other in much more than a physical sense. They must try to understand each other's emotional needs and strive to meet them. The couple will be interested in each other's values, goals, and ideas and will share spiritual insights. Only then can they truly "know" each other sufficiently to join their bodies in a complete knowing. And since the years will change their feelings, ideas, and perhaps even their interests, such knowing each other must be a continuous process of communicating and sharing.

Being increasingly able to participate in this type of openness can lead to a higher sense of intimacy. A couple who have only physical proximity of bodies without the other components of togetherness cannot be considered truly intimate. Intimacy denotes a closeness of the whole person.

This type of experience reflects the meaning of the word "within." When married lovers are "within" each other's life boundaries, they are sharing at a level unique to the marital relationship, a space not open to others.

The beautiful part is that when God is central in our lives, He can revive flagging or even troubled marriages. Through God's abiding love we receive the power to love each other as He has loved us.

ALBERTA MAZAT

*Dear Father, we know that we can't manufacture love on our own. But we praise You for the promise that You can love through us. Amen.*

# Think Happy, Feel Better

*Whatever is true, whatever is noble, whatever is right, whatever is pure, whatever is lovely, whatever is admirable—if anything is excellent or praiseworthy—think about such things. Phil. 4:8, NIV.*

**D**id you know that . . .
• Socially active married people tend to live longer than less active separated, divorced, or single people? And happily married women have the strongest immune systems of all?

• Men who participate in social activities at least once a week outlive men who don't?

• Confiding in someone else can result in a significant improvement in immune-system function?

• Those men who were most pessimistic at age 25 had more severe illness during their 40s, 50s, and 60s?

• There is a relationship between psychological factors and susceptibility to colds—i.e., pessimists are more likely to get colds?

• Even thinking about love can raise the level of salivary immunoglobulin A in some individuals?

• When patients were trained to focus on the

positive aspects of their postsurgery hospital stay, they used only half as many painkillers and stayed in the hospital an average of two days less than others?

The brain and the immune system have a strong linkage. For example, Donald Robinson tells of a long-term study reported in the prestigious British medical journal *The Lancet* on 57 breast cancer victims that had undergone mastectomies. Seventy percent of the women who had a "fighting spirit" were alive 10 years later compared to only 20 percent of the women who "felt hopeless." Three fourths of those who merely accepted their diagnosis also died.

In 1987 Candace Pert, while at the National Institute of Mental Health, suggested a molecular equivalent of telephone lines between the brain and the immune system by which white blood cells receive messages directly from the brain to fight off disease invaders.

What message is your brain sending to your immune system? Is it any wonder that God inspired the apostle Paul to instruct us to think about things that were true, noble, right, pure, lovely, admirable, excellent, and praiseworthy?

JAN W. AND KAY KUZMA

*Dear Lord, help me to focus on the positive and spend time with my friends and family.*

# The Cleansing Power

*If we confess our sins, He is faithful and just to forgive us our sins and to cleanse us from all unrighteousness. 1 John 1:9, NKJV.*

The summer heat was already intensifying as I stood and stretched my aching muscles. Even at 9:00 a.m. the July sun was potent. I had learned that the never-ending work of maintaining a yard was best done early in the day. Wiping the sweat from my face, I smiled at the results of this morning's work. The flower bed was again rid of those noxious, prickly thistles. It looked pretty good, though I couldn't take credit for the rainbow array of perennial flowers that brightened our landscape. The previous owner had shown a real talent for arranging and planning flower beds that would complement the uneven terrain. My job was to try to keep the weeds removed.

Returning the gardening tools to the garage, I gratefully headed for the shower. The dust and dirt of the garden mixed with sweat might be a sign of honest labor, but it was hardly a thing to cherish longer than necessary. As the warm water and soap removed the unpleasant aroma of my morning's toil, I thanked the Lord again for the convenience of abundant hot water and modern plumbing. Not only did the soap and water remove the dirt, but they also brought relief to muscles unaccustomed to such agricultural pursuits.

When God created the skin to cover the human body, He could have made it as tough as that of the turtle's shell. Instead our skin is supple, strong, and so sensitive that, according to Paul Brand and Philip Yancey in *Fearfully and Wonderfully Made*, we can discern a thousandth of an ounce of pressure on the tip of a half inch of hair. No wonder the warm spray of a shower is so delightfully refreshing!

Rejuvenated, I stepped from the shower ready to tackle the rest of the day's tasks. The psalmist had recognized the restorative power of water when he prayed, "Wash away all my iniquity and cleanse me from my sin. . . . Cleanse me with hyssop, and I will be clean; wash me, and I will be whiter than snow" (Ps. 51:2-7, NIV).

ROSE SHAFER FULLER

*Thank You, Lord, that Your cleansing water of life is even more available than the warm water in my shower. Please wash me every day.*

# In My Most Embarrassing Moments

*But he said to me, "My grace is sufficient for you, for my power is made perfect in weakness." 2 Cor. 12:9, NIV.*

Father, today I tried to take out my patient's teeth to wash, only to discover that they weren't dentures. One of my confused patients thought his water pitcher was a urinal, and I ordered two meal trays for the same patient and both were the wrong diet.

That's not all.

I embarrassed myself by asking my patient's wife if she was his daughter. The student nurse asked me a simple question, and I didn't know the answer.

Days like this make me feel inadequate. Help me, Father, not to be critical of myself.

Remind me that Your followers of old had days like this too. Peter failed at walking on water and Jonah jumped into the belly of a whale.

Their "bad" days passed. Mine will too.

Do your prayers sometimes sound like mine? Do you sometimes have days when nothing seems to go right? You get up early and have a neat devotional time with the Lord, get dressed in your new outfit, and head off to work, thinking the day will be great, only to end up getting a traffic ticket on the street all your colleagues take coming to work. Or at the end of the day find the sales tag still on the jacket you've been wearing!

I'm convinced that sometimes I'm more the bull in a china closet trying to get through the day than a neurosurgeon cauterizing tiny blood vessels in the brain. My blundering ways cause more embarrassment than I care to endure.

That's why I need that devotional time with the Lord. God can't keep me from making a fool of myself, but He can remind me each morning that even though He lives in a high and holy place and will never make a mistake, He lives with those who do—"with him who is contrite and lowly in spirit, *to revive the spirit of the lowly and to revive the heart of the contrite*" (Isa. 57:15, NIV).

Many days I am contrite—broken, crushed—and need a heart revived by God.

CARLA GOBER

*Thank You, Father, for Your daily reminder that You will never laugh at my mistakes, but will proudly stand by my side in my most embarrassing moments.*

# Are You a Ten-Talent Cook?

*She gets up while it is still dark; she provides food for her family. . . . Give her the reward she has earned, and let her works bring her praise at the city gate. Prov. 31:15-31, NIV.*

Often health reform is made health deform by unpalatable preparation of food. The lack of knowledge regarding healthful cookery must be remedied before health reform is a success.

"Good cooks are few. Many, many mothers need to take lessons in cooking, that they may set before the family well-prepared, neatly served food.

"Before children take lessons on the organ or the piano they should be given lessons in cooking. The work of learning to cook need not exclude music, but to learn music is of less importance than to learn how to prepare food that is wholesome and appetizing. . . .

"It is a sin to place poorly prepared food on the table, because the matter of eating concerns the well-being of the entire system. The Lord desires His people to appreciate the necessity of having food prepared in such a way that it will not make sour stomachs and in consequence sour tempers. Let us remember that there is practical religion in a loaf of good bread.

"Let not the work of cooking be looked upon as a sort of slavery. What would become of those in our world if all who are engaged in cooking should give up their work with the flimsy excuse that it is not sufficiently dignified? Cooking may be regarded as less desirable than some other lines of work, but in reality it is a science above all other sciences. Thus God regards the preparation of healthful food. He places a high estimate on those who do faithful service in preparing wholesome, palatable food.

"The one who understands the art of properly preparing food, and who uses this knowledge, is worthy of higher commendation than those engaged in any other line of work. This talent should be regarded as equal in value to ten talents; for its right use has much to do with keeping the human organism in health. Because so inseparably connected with life and health, it is the most valuable of all gifts" (*Medical Ministry*, pp. 270, 271).

"The foundation of that which keeps people in health is the medical missionary work of good cooking" (*ibid.*, p. 270).

ELLEN G. WHITE

*What could you do to enhance your cooking skills?*

# Staying Fit

*I am the vine; you are the branches. If a man remains in me and I in him, he will bear much fruit; apart from me you can do nothing. John 15:5, NIV.*

When it comes to our bodies, nothing lasts forever. First we are young, then we grow old. After eating a meal, we get hungry again. We drink to our fill, but need more water later. And no matter how much we exercise to stay in shape, that effect wears off if we do not repeat it regularly.

Experts in exercise physiology tell us that the body starts to decondition after 48 hours of nonactivity. That means if you rest too long between exercise sessions, your body will begin to lose its tone. If you neglect exercise long enough, you will eventually lose most of the benefits of your previous efforts.

I learned that lesson myself with great frustration one year when a knee injury forced me to suspend my jogging routine for several months. Prior to this injury, I was averaging 20 miles a week. After my recuperation I returned to the track and could barely run a mile without feeling winded. It was a discouraging setback and a painful reminder to me that exercise must be continual for the benefits to linger. I cannot take this year off and expect last year's efforts to carry me on indefinitely.

When it comes to my relationship with God, the rules are very much the same. A healthy Christian experience requires a regular routine of prayer, study, and connection with our heavenly Father. Like eating, sleeping, and exercising, it demands daily attention. And like our physical bodies, our spiritual vitality quickly atrophies with indolence.

God could have designed us to draw all our nutrition by simply breathing the required nutrients from the air around us. Then we wouldn't have to deal with the daily necessity of eating. He could have engineered our physiology so that a one-mile jog would yield Olympic results for a lifetime. But He didn't, and I suspect He had a reason, with a lesson to teach us.

Human physical and spiritual requirements are similar. Ignore your body's needs, and you pay a price in weakness and debilitation. Neglect your relationship with God, and your spiritual health will wither like a branch cut off from the vine.

So, get fit—but don't forget to *stay* fit.

LARRY RICHARDSON

*It's time to get organized. What in your physical or spiritual life should you schedule into your day, to make sure you stay fit?*

# When You Feel
# a Worry Coming On

*You will keep in perfect peace him whose mind is steadfast, because he trusts in you. Isa. 26:3, NIV.*

Lyndon B. Johnson, former president of the United States, once told an audience in Stonewall, Texas, that he was feeling fine because he had followed the advice of an old woman who once said, "When I walks, I walks slowly. When I sits, I sits loosely. And when I feels worry comin' on, I just goes to sleep." That old woman was not a psychologist, but she gave great advice to those who live in a high-tech, high-stress world plagued with depression, worry, and anxiety.

First, "When I walks, I walks slowly." In other words, don't rush through life. Slow down enough to enjoy the scenery and stop to smell the flowers along the way.

Second, "When I sits, I sits loosely." Don't get too comfortable with what you have, who you are, or what you do. Life is difficult, and sometimes circumstances beyond your control can rip your security away and force change upon you. It's best to be flexible in times like this. As those in the West Indies say, "Hang loose, mon"!

And third, "When I feels worry comin' on, I just goes to sleep." Sleep is a great battery charger. As life falls apart and you don't think you can cope, one of the best things you can do is get some sleep. Things always look brighter in the morning!

God has some great advice too. Read again Jesus' words in Matthew 6:27-35. Why do you worry, since if God takes care of little things such as birds and flowers, He can take care of you even more? All He asks you to do is live one day at a time.

Peter underscores this same message in 1 Peter 5:7, in which he says we should give our cares to God. Letting go and allowing Christ to take care of you and your problems isn't as easy as it sounds if you're used to fixing things yourself. But God says if you'll just trust in Him, He'll give you perfect peace. Why not give it a try?

CAROLINE WATKINS

*Give all your worries to the Lord and trust that He will answer your prayers, and He will give you perfect peace.*

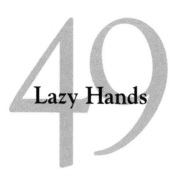

# Lazy Hands

*Lazy hands make a man poor, but diligent hands bring wealth.*
Prov. 10:4, NIV.

After an automobile accident in 1972, I missed my freshman year of high school. But I loved the physical therapy I had to take, and during that year I worked so hard that my therapist told me *he* needed a rest! You see, I knew the harder I worked, the sooner I'd walk out of there and back to school.

Nobody told me I had a badly damaged spinal cord. It probably wouldn't have mattered anyway, because I was very stubborn. I remember thinking that a broken neck is like a broken arm or leg. They heal, and everything gets back to normal. Sometimes ignorance is bliss.

The next year I went back to school—but not walking. I'd regained feeling and a little movement, however, on my left side. I had begun my life right-handed, but now I was an unwilling southpaw. I could sign my name, mark T or F, circle multiple-choice answers, borrow classmates' notes, and take

103

essay exams orally. Did I really need to learn to write?

Yes, according to my English teacher. Mr. Jones told our class we had to write a one-page essay a day. I thought I'd get an extra 10 minutes to read, study, or whatever. Not so. When I said I couldn't write without a table, he said to use his desk. And when I said I couldn't write a page, he told me to compose three or four lines. I couldn't talk my way out of this one. So I wrote and I wrote—and I hated it. If Jones and I hadn't been friends, I don't know how things would have turned out.

With Jones's discipline, the care he had for me, and God's continuing gift of healing, I began writing with my left hand. If God hadn't cared about my writing, and Jones hadn't allowed God to use him, it's highly unlikely I'd be sharing this with you today.

I know that we can all do more than we think we can, *if we don't give up*, and we give God a chance to work out His will for us in our lives.

THERESE L. ALLEN

*Have you been putting off learning a skill or doing something you've never done before because it's hard work? Why not start today to put in the extra effort needed for God to work out His will in your life?*

# A Lesson in Hope
## and Healing

*May the God of hope fill you with all joy and peace as you trust in him, so that you may overflow with hope by the power of the Holy Spirit. Rom. 15:13, NIV.*

Children with cancer certainly have much to feel discouraged and hopeless about. Daily they suffer many painful experiences, and the side effects of chemotherapy and other treatments affect their body image and self-esteem. Yet most children and adolescents with cancer face their situations with a positive outlook and cheerfulness that amazes those who work with them. I believe the key is their faith and hope in the future.

Ann is an example of this. She was diagnosed with sarcoma at the age of 13, then treated with radical surgery, radiation, and two years of chemotherapy. With no relapses for more than 10 years, she is now classified as a long-term survivor.

Rather than blaming God for her illness, Ann saw Him as the source of her strength. Her faith in God grew stronger through her therapy. As a result of her experiences undergoing treatment for cancer, she made a decision to dedicate her life to helping others. She is now enrolled in graduate study in medical ethics and plans to become a hospital chaplain.

Ann acutely believes her experience as a cancer patient was the most positive experience of her life. She is convinced her faith and hope enabled her to become a survivor. As she expressed it: "I believe the experience fundamentally changed who I am. I value life more. I take joy in the little things, like the smell of a flower or the color of a sunset. I think a lot of people make their own lives difficult. Each of us needs to enjoy each day God gives us."

Whenever I feel overwhelmed or discouraged by the stresses and problems of my life, I think of Ann. I am simply unable to feel sorry for myself when I reflect on her courage. Her life is a powerful lesson in hope and healing.

With God's help, we, like Ann, can learn to view all of life's experiences as positive. If we let Him, God can turn the bad things that happen to us into positive things that strengthen our faith, deepen our trust in Him, and fill us with joy and hope.

LINDA WILLMAN JOHNSON

*Make Romans 15:13 your personal prayer: "May the God of hope fill me, [your name], with all joy and peace as I trust in Him, so that I may overflow with hope by the power of the Holy Spirit."*

# For What
# Do You Strive?

*I will not leave you as orphans; I will come to you. Before long, the world will not see me anymore, but you will see me. Because I live, you also will live. On that day you will realize that I am in my Father, and you are in me, and I am in you. John 14:18-20, NIV.*

It made no sense. He'd spent four years diligently turning himself from an overweight, heavy-smoking, hypertensive borderline alcoholic into an almost physically fit individual. He scheduled himself and his wife for comprehensive physical evaluations from which he received an excellent report. Physically he was in the best shape he'd been in for years. Eight weeks later, under the pressure of financial reverses, he thrust a knife into his chest and died.

Here was a man who'd worked so hard to please *somebody*—maybe a parent, maybe himself, maybe a God he didn't understand. I had the task of preparing records for the insurance adjusters that required me to review each entry in his chart over the past 10 years. That, with a small degree of personal knowledge of him, created a haunting picture in my mind of a terribly lonely person. He must have had some unattainable image of what he must be, what he must do, and what he must obtain and maintain in life in order to be acceptable.

Most of us have experienced loneliness and the desire for acceptance. For some it's a transient thing brought on by circumstances like moving or the loss of a loved one. For others it's a gnawing need that eats at the very core of their existence. It seems that nothing can satisfy until they meet the demands of that emotional core.

God has an answer to meet even this. Do you long for a father's love? Read Jeremiah 31:3, NIV: "I have loved you with an everlasting love; I have drawn you with loving-kindness." Do you miss a mother's love? Read Isaiah 49:15, NIV: "Can a mother forget the baby at her breast and have no compassion on the child she has borne?" Claim this love as your own—for it truly is.

Then examine your life. Is what you are doing an effort to gain acceptance? Or is it because you are God's and you are accepted and loved, and you are availing yourself of privileged opportunities?

LOIS (RITTENHOUSE) PECCE

*Are you aggressive and fearless on the outside, but hurting and empty inside? Open that pain to Jesus. He waits for you with love.*

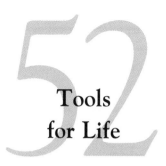

# Tools
# for Life

*Sing and make music in your heart to the Lord, always giving thanks to God the Father for everything, in the name of our Lord Jesus Christ. Eph. 5:19, 20, NIV.*

Like many women, I grew up believing that if I was a very good girl, followed all the rules, and loved God enough, life would turn out pretty well. What a disappointment, therefore, to wake up one morning in adulthood to discover that the formula had failed. My health had taken a decided dip. I was a walking combination of burnout, disappointment, frustration, and midlife crisis.

In frustration I turned to a more in-depth study of the brain and the immune system. Emerging research provided some practical tools that changed my life. For example, I learned that although we often use the terms *emotions* and *feelings* interchangeably, they are not the same. Emotions arise in the brain's limbic system (pain-pleasure center) and are simply little flags designed to get our attention. Information about the physiological changes these emotions cause in the body travels to the cerebrum (thinking portion of the brain). There we assign weight to these flags, and our interpretations then become our feelings.

Practically, this means that while we may not always have complete control over our initial emotions, within six or seven seconds of becoming aware of our thoughts we can begin to take control of our feelings.

First I learned to identify the entire range of emotions God has placed in the human brain. Next I honed the ability to translate those flags into feelings more accurately. Gradually I gave myself permission to feel all my feelings until eventually I accepted complete responsibility for managing my emotions and feelings.

Often we handle them with faulty screens we have absorbed early in life. I actually did some very helpful family-of-origin work to discover some of the generationally transmitted response patterns that had been operating among the members of my family.

The bottom line? If we want to change the way we feel, we need to change the way we think. It is our choice to maintain a giving feeling, to choose a different feeling, or to act upon a feeling, thus moving us from a position of helplessness toward one of empowerment.

ARLENE TAYLOR

*What steps can you take to manage your emotions and feelings more successfully? Are you allowing your brain to be God-educated and Holy Spirit-impressed?*

# Out of the Ashes of My Life

*To appoint unto them that mourn in Zion, to give unto them beauty for ashes, the oil of joy for mourning, the garment of praise for the spirit of heaviness; that they might be called trees of righteousness, the planting of the Lord, that he might be glorified. Isa. 61:3.*

How many times had I been the one listening to the heartbreak of a wife going through a divorce she never dreamed would happen? Now it had happened to me! The shock and disbelief left me numb. My mind reeled as I tried to sort out this cataclysmic emotional trauma from the already heavy pressures of wife, mother, daughter, worker, and church and community volunteer. Dad was ailing and nearing death. Mother was trying to be courageous after a recent leg amputation. Both needed loving support and care. I felt as David did when he mournfully sang, "Faint and badly crushed I groan aloud in anguish of heart" (Ps. 38:8, REB).

Broken under the weight of it all, I staggered outdoors into the mild August evening air. There I found myself in the midst of my vegetable garden, furiously weeding the bean patch. Each clump of weeds felt like an enemy evicted. As I stepped back to view the weeded row with a sense of satisfaction and relief, a sudden pleasing aroma surrounded me. Wondering about its source, I glanced downward. In disbelief I realized I had trampled on my basil plants!

Standing motionless as the quiet fragrance enveloped me, I was impressed that it took "crushing" and "brokenness" to produce the sudden fragrance that had proved such a blessed experience.

Yes, Christ's body was broken for *me* and sin crushed Him, bringing forth the fragrant gift of salvation for *me!* With a deeply thankful heart I prayerfully walked from the garden, nurtured by the object lesson that God could take my "crushed" and "broken" life and make me a fragrance for Him.

After my divorce, while my friends were retiring from work, I found myself enrolled in graduate school, prayerfully pursuing a master's degree in public health. During this same time a prayer band was praying for someone to start a van ministry in Boston. A week after my graduation the Boston Van Ministry was born out of the ashes of my life, perfumed with crushed basil!

J. RITA VITAL

*When you feel broken and crushed, remember that God has promised beauty for ashes!*

# 54

# Tap Into God's
# Water Supply

*For I will pour water on the thirsty land, and streams on the dry ground; I will pour out my Spirit on your offspring, and my blessing on your descendants. Isa. 44:3, NIV.*

It all started when mountaineering teams from several nations sought to be the first to conquer Mount Everest, the tallest mountain in the world. The elite Swiss team, considered by many to be the best, made the first attempt, but failed.

A year later, in 1953, the British decided to try. As they carefully studied the records of the Swiss expedition, they made an interesting discovery. The Swiss team members drank less than two glasses of water each day. Could that be the reason for their failure? Consequently, the British climbers ordered extra snow-melting equipment. The men drank 12 glasses of water a day, and they reached the top!

Most people underestimate the amount of water they lose while active. Some athletes lose up to five quarts. If you don't replace this lost fluid, not only do you feel severe fatigue, but you lose essential salts as well. If you wait until you feel thirsty, that's too late.

Your body is already suffering from dehydration and symptoms of exhaustion.

Water is nature's energy source on tap. It can help you get your house painted or your lawn mowed. The vital fluid gives you energy to finish that marathon you never thought you could run, or climb a mountain peak!

But water can do more than that. Have you ever visited Palm Springs? On one lot you'll see nothing but sand and desert brush, and right next to it grow lush green grass, shady palms, and flowers of every variety. What makes the difference? Water.

God's Spirit is a lot like water. When it comes into people the change is dramatic. Energy, motivations, and talents blossom into life. People now have power to say no to habits that have held them captive for years. They have strength to conquer mountains of guilt and confusion that had seemed hopeless. But just as a few days without water turns the garden into a desert, so it is with us. So for best results, drink freely of God's Spirit throughout the day.

NANCY NEWBALL

*Drink eight glasses of water today, even if you don't feel like it. The results will far outweigh your efforts.*

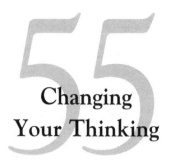

# Changing
# Your Thinking

*Search me, O God, and know my heart; test me and know my anxious thoughts. See if there is any offensive way in me, and lead me in the way everlasting. Ps. 139:23, 24, NIV.*

A fundamental law of psychological well-being is that *you become what you think you are.* Your thoughts are incredible motivators as your thinking shapes your behavior. Therefore, it is vitally important to guard the avenues of your mind so you don't allow Satan to flood you with guilt, discouragement, anxiety, and depression.

Here's a five-step plan to safeguard your mind from Satan's attacks.

First, develop the habit of thinking of good things—interesting things: your successes, achievements, opportunities for service, people in need whose lives you can brighten.

Second, develop the habit of looking at every problem and difficulty as a stepping-stone to victory. I have never forgotten the cartoon of a boy with a saw looking with dismay at a piece of board with a notch he had just cut out to fit around a post. It was obvious he had cut out the wrong side of the board, but I'll never forget the caption: "Even a mistake shows you've tried!" Look at every mistake as something you can profit from—a stepping-stone to victory.

Third, feel yourself toughening up the muscles of your character as you tackle the unpleasant tasks, the mundane chores, the messy jobs. And then take as your motto, "I'll always be true to my conscience."

Fourth, make a habit of smiling at people from the inside. Practice feeling your happy thoughts toward the people you meet.

Fifth, memorize key scriptural promises that can carry you through periods of discouragement or despondency. Here are three:

• "The righteous cry out, and the Lord hears them; he delivers them from all their troubles. The Lord is close to the brokenhearted and saves those who are crushed in spirit" (Ps. 34:17, 18, NIV).

• "Blessed is the man who perseveres under trial, because when he has stood the test, he will receive the crown of life that God has promised to those who love him" (James 1:12, NIV).

• "Be strong and courageous. Do not be terrified; do not be discouraged, for the Lord your God will be with you wherever you go" (Joshua 1:9, NIV).

ELDEN M. CHALMERS

*Ask God to help you hold on to the promises in Psalm 34:17, 18; James 1:12; and Joshua 1:9 and to give you victory over your discouraging and anxious thoughts.*

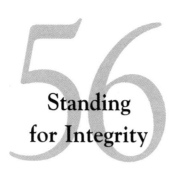

# Standing for Integrity

*Because the Sovereign Lord helps me, I will not be disgraced. Therefore have I set my face like flint, and I know I will not be put to shame. Isa. 50:7, NIV.*

Thomas More is well known as one of the great moral and ethical heroes of the Western world, and each of us lives his story in microcosm in the daily decisions we face.

The great question of his life was how to respond to the divorce and remarriage of King Henry VIII. Frustrated by her inability to produce a male heir, Henry divorced Catherine of Aragon and married Anne Boleyn. The church opposed the divorce and delayed approving the new marriage. Henry put pressure on Parliament to pass the act of succession to transfer the royal lineage from the children of Catherine to the children of Anne.

The members of Parliament, with various degrees of enthusiasm, ultimately went along, with one exception—Thomas More.

More paid a high price for his faithfulness to principle.

His reputation for integrity was well known. More's approval would have helped to silence the king's conscience, but his refusal to go along pricked the king's comfort and disturbed his peace.

The king had More confined in a filthy dungeon and his income cut off. His wife and daughter were reduced to poverty. England watched and the king waited for More's signature approving the act of succession.

More held out for two years, but his wife lost all patience with his unyieldingly principled life.

Tradition says that someone entered his filthy cell and found More surrounded by vagabonds, brigands, thieves, and killers. The gentle scholar sat emaciated, clad in rags, shivering from the cold. The visitor had brought the list of parliamentary signatures, signatures of friends and companions from law and life. He begged More to sign and save his life: "But Thomas, look at these names. You know these men. Can't you do what I did, and come with us, for fellowship?"

More responded: "And when we stand before God, and you are sent to heaven for doing according to your conscience and I am sent to hell for not doing according to mine, will you come with me for fellowship?"

M. JERRY DAVIS

*Are you living according to God's principles, or do you find yourself compromising when tempted? Think about More's response.*

# Health Is Wholeness

*Do you not know that your body is a temple of the Holy Spirit, who is in you, whom you have received from God? You are not your own; you were bought at a price. Therefore honor God with your body. 1 Cor. 6:19, 20, NIV.*

One of the major myths in modern society is the passion for fitness as an end in itself. I have a friend who is totally caught up in the fitness craze, working out at a fitness palace virtually every night. Vitamins and supplements that promise to give her greater energy and help her eliminate deposits of fat (of which a casual look would suggest she has few) clutter her desk. She subscribes to body-building magazines that display sculptured bodies that seem almost inhuman in the extremes of muscle definition. She even had dreams of competing in such contests herself.

On the surface it would seem that she has a passion for health. Surely, trying to look good and feel good are positive things. But health is more than muscle definition. And fitness is more than the relationship between weight and body fat.

In her pursuit of the perfect body, my friend has

chosen to exclude from her life many other elements that contribute to overall wholeness. Her marriages have ended painfully, and the relationship she's in now is quite unconventional. She has selected for her preferred social setting the bars and clubs that cater to the mindless, pleasure-seeking crowd, most of which is a generation younger than she is. She no longer attends church or finds anything appealing in the spiritual dimension of life.

The real problem with what she is doing, however, isn't so much the elements she's brought into her life (though others might choose differently), but the elements she's excluded. A life in balance is one that places the physical aspect in proper perspective with the others, including the social, the intellectual, and the spiritual. Health is wholeness, a life in which all the parts work together in a symmetry that exceeds just that of a sculpted body. And in so doing, we honor God with our bodies, not self.

I know "man does not live on bread alone" (Matt. 4:4, NIV) but it must also be said that we should not live by exercise alone, either!

DAN DAY

*Remember that "holiness is wholeness for God; it is the entire surrender of heart and life to the indwelling of the principles of heaven"* (The Desire of Ages, *p. 556*).

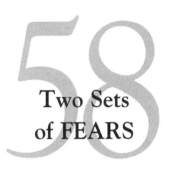

# Two Sets
# of FEARS

*For God has not given us a spirit of fear, but of power and of love and of a sound mind. 2 Tim. 1:7, NKJV.*

Seven-year-old Laurie, clinging to her mother's arm, eyed her pediatrician like a scared rabbit. Mother had brought her to see the doctor because she had been vomiting for the past four weeks. It had begun the day after Labor Day. The doctor was quick to discover that the day after Labor Day had been the day Laurie had started school for the first time. Thrust into a new situation that filled her with fear, she had developed an anxiety that had sent nerve impulses that tightened her stomach, causing her to vomit.

Adults also suffer from fear and anxiety, manifested by a variety of feelings. Some of the main ones we can describe by the acronym FEARS: Frustration, Envy, Anger, Resentment, and Sadness. These negative feelings cause changes in various organs in our body. They influence the amount of blood that flows to an organ. When we are embarrassed, for example, our face and neck turn red. As too much blood rushes to the head, headache may result.

Stress affects the heart. Repressed hostility has been associated with heart attacks. Also, stress can elevate the level of adrenal hormones—epinephrine and corticosteroid—which can raise the blood pressure as well as suppress the immune system. In addition, stress affects the muscles, causing neck tension and back pain, and the gastrointestinal and nervous systems as well.

To overcome stress we can use the same acronym, FEARS. F is for Faith in God—we need to trust God, who knows all our troubles. Exercise, both physical and spiritual, is crucial. We need Acceptance of ourselves and others. "Be kindly affectioned one to another with brotherly love; in honour preferring one another" (Rom. 12:10). R stands for Rest—not only physical rest but also the rest Jesus is so willing to give us (Matt. 11:28). S is for Singing. When your spirit is low, take a short walk and sing a chorus such as "Jesus, loving Jesus, sweetest name I know, fills my ev'ry longing, keeps me singing as I go." We need not fear when we have Jesus.

BENJAMIN LAU

*What FEARS do you have? The first set: Frustration, Envy, Anger, Resentment, and Sadness; or the second set: Faith, Exercise, Acceptance, Rest, and Singing?*

# Of Lightbulbs and Health

*You are the light of the world. A city on a hill cannot be hidden. Neither do people light a lamp and put it under a bowl. Instead they put it on its stand, and it gives light to everyone . . . , let your light shine before men, that they may see your good deeds and praise your Father. Matt. 5:14-16, NIV.*

Yesterday I ran into Mr. Ultrahealth. Thirty-one years of age, committed to a daily one-hour workout on his Nautilus machine, he is in fabulous shape. His hobby is rock-climbing and his diet consists of piles of unsprayed fruits and vegetables, mounds of alfalfa sprouts, and barrels of oat bran. He drinks 10 glasses of distilled water a day, sleeps eight hours at night, regards sweets with utter disdain, and never forgets to floss his teeth. In addition, his cholesterol is below 130, he has never been in a hospital, and his physician says he has never seen anybody healthier.

Today, however, I saw him kick the dog, scream obscenities at his wife, and leave the house without saying goodbye to his children. At work he lied to his boss, blaming a colleague for his own mistake. He was unkind, impatient, selfish, immoral, and spiritually bankrupt.

And suddenly a light came on in my mind.

Health is more than eating right and exercising daily. Fitness involves more than first meets the eye. Actually, health is more like a lightbulb. The glass may be shiny, clean, and clear on the outside. But if the filament on the inside is broken or disconnected from the core, then there won't be any light. Yet without light the bulb will have missed its purpose.

Lightbulbs aren't ends in themselves. They're only a means to an end, only valuable if they help us get to where we really want to go.

As we look forward to the new year, let us take a closer look at our goal of health. If our lifestyle improvements don't help us to become more loving persons, then we are as worthless as a broken lightbulb. We may look polished on the outside, but without being connected on the inside we are not bringing light to others.

The ultimate purpose of pursuing health remains to become a more efficient lightbulb—to serve others better.

HANS DIEHL

*Lord, may my life shine with love to others. Amen.*

# Promises—Promises

*Watch and pray so that you will not fall into temptation. The spirit is willing, but the body is weak. Matt. 26:41, NIV.*

One of the most common New Year's resolutions is in the area of health—either to lose weight, change our diet, or exercise more. Psychologically the new year seems an appropriate time to make a new start, and so we all vow to be better in some way.

Health clubs around the country swell with new memberships every January. You can hardly find a free StairMaster or cycling machine. Aerobics classes are jam-packed. Sporting good stores love the month of January. They sell sweat suits, running shoes, and exercise equipment by the truckload to all the New Year's health converts. January clients besiege weight-loss clinics everywhere. And bookstores brace for a run on health, diet, and fitness books after the new year.

For the first few weeks of the new year we make good on our promise to turn our lives around, for "the spirit" is indeed willing and seems to fuel our determination. But soon reality sets in and "the flesh" begins to rebel. We find that breaking old lifestyle habits is not as easy as a New Year's promise and a brand-new running suit. We begin to invent excuses to neglect our resolution: "It's too cold outside." "It's too late today." "I'm too tired." "My toe hurts." "I'll do it tomorrow." "This isn't fun anymore." And so on. By February we have pretty much returned to our old routines. The health clubs are once again ghost towns, and those brand-new running shoes get lost in the closet.

Jesus summed up the human condition with His memorable quote for today, and He should know, for He shared our frailties while here on earth. But He also showed us that our true source of strength lies not in our own feeble willpower, but in joining forces with divinity.

So, if you have faltered on New Year's resolutions in the past, remember: "I can do all things through Christ who strengthens me" (Phil. 4:13, NKJV) and lace up those walking shoes for a healthy new year.

LARRY RICHARDSON

*Make three resolutions for a healthy new year and pray this prayer: "Lord, give me Your strength to keep the resolutions I have made, for my spirit is willing, but my flesh is weak. Amen."*

Books by Jan W. Kuzma,
Kay Kuzma, and DeWitt S. Williams:

*60 Ways to Energize Your Life*
*Energized!*

To order, **call 1-800-765-6955.**

**Vist us at www.rhpa.org** for more information
on Review and Herald products.

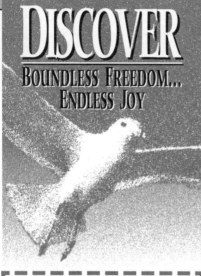